A Patient's Guide

A Healthy Diet to Heal Nerve Pain

Dr. Bao Thai, DC

ISBN-10: 1975720075

ISBN-13: 978-1975720070

Dedication

I wanted to sincerely thank everyone that has made this possible, especially my staff and my family. Without all of your support, my vision would never come true.

To Suzanne and Connor,

You are my driving force and what keeps me working so hard to help other people. Without you, I would not be the person I am today.

Table of Contents

Section 1 6

   Nerve Damage & Pain...6

   Types of Nerve Pain 7

   Diseases That Cause Nerve Pain 9

   Types of Nerve Pain 10

Section 2 13

   How to Treat Nerve Pain..13

Section 3 17

   How A Poor Diet Affects Your Happiness 17

   What is a Poor Diet? 18

   Consequences of a Poor Diet..20

   Steps for Improving your Diet...25

Section 4 28

   What is wrong with the food we eat? 28

Section 5 33

   What is the impact of the food we eat? 33

Section 6 39

   How Pharmaceutical Drugs Affect People with a Poor Diet ..39

Section 7 44

   The Ramifications of Poor Nutrition and Consuming Pain
   Killers 44

Section 8 51

   20 Miraculous Foods That Can Reverse Nerve Damage and
   Reduce Pain 51

   Herbs That Can Reverse Nerve Damage and Reduce Pain.....57

Section 9 60

  Recipes...60

Section 1

Nerve Damage & Pain

Like your digestive system, you always need a perfectly working nervous system to maintain your health. The nervous system is comprised of the central nervous system and the peripheral nervous system. The central nervous system consists of the brain and spinal cord, whereas the peripheral nervous system is comprised of everything outside of your brain and spinal cord.

The nerves play a vital role in making the nervous system work. Nerves, in simple words, are like the branches of a tree transferring messages from your body to the trunk - the brain and the spinal cord. These nerves contain receptors that sense stimuli from the external environment, send the received message to the brain which then send the message to the specified organ to bring about a response.

For example, when you touch a sharp needle, you would certainly want to move your hand from it quickly. This is possible when the nerves and specialized cells called neurons receive a stimulus and take that message to the central nervous system.

The central nervous system sends the message back so an appropriate muscle response can be made to move the hand from the pointed pin to get rid of the pain. This seems like a simple process where nerves work without any hassle at all. But this can be complicated as well, especially when one experiences nerve pain or nerve damage.

Nerve pain is a state that may be experienced at any time of the day or night, either continuously or intermittently. If you wake up in the middle of night experiencing a chronic burning, tingling or immense prickling sensation that is difficult to bear, you must be aware that this nerve pain needs to be treated as soon as possible.

Nerve pain in the feet is very common. One may experience nerve pain in the feet due to a problem in the lower spine or from a problem between the spinal cord and the feet. Other parts of the body can also have extreme nerve pain similar to that in the feet.

The case of nerve damage is a bit different than nerve pain and it can be even more dangerous, as it causes numbness which can be deadly. Nerve damage can occur to the nerves in your central nervous system. The brain and spinal cord, and any nerve in the peripheral nervous system, may be a victim of this damage.

Nerve damage causes numbness, so you might not sense pain. There are so many nuances that it is often over looked as the serious the problem it actually is.

Types of Nerve Pain

There are three different types of nerves: autonomic, motor, and sensory. All are prone to damage, though differently, and that nerve pain can result from multiple known and unknown causes. Experts do not restrict it to just a tingling feeling or numbness.

There are some general all-encompassing symptoms that are associated with nerve damage.

- Pain

- Sensitivity

- Prickling and tingling

- Numbness

- Burning

- Weakness

- Muscle weakness

- Sweating disorder (Too much or too little)

- Twitching

- Paralysis

- Constipation

- Dry eyes and dry mouth

- Bladder dysfunction

- Sexual dysfunction

These symptoms may occur independently or in combination with others. Most of the time, when two or more of these symptoms occur together, it means more than one nerve is damaged.

Diseases That Cause Nerve Pain

While nerve pain and nerve damage can be a side effect of drugs and trauma, there are some diseases that can cause nerve pain and nerve damage on top of other symptoms.

Autoimmune Disease

According to the American Autoimmune Related Diseases Association (AARDA), 50% of Americans suffer from this type of disease, where the immune system attacks the peripheral nervous system causing nerve pain and damage.

Cancer

Chemotherapy is a very common cause of nerve damage. The medication starts to break down the outer lining of the nerve, thus exposing it. Chemotherapy is a toxin that is designed to destroy cancer cells. The problem is that it destroys all cells in the process, including nerves.

Diabetes

Over 50% of diabetic patients will suffer from neuropathy according to the American Diabetic Association. The body's inability to control glucose properly will cause excess inflammation. The inflammation will lead to the breakdown of the nerves in the body. The end result is nerve damage.

Trauma

Trauma is one of the leading causes of nerve pain. It can compress the nerves resulting in deadly nerve pain and damage. Trauma can be from an accident or the result of surgery. It is very common for a patient to have nerve damage as result of spinal surgery.

HIV

One third of people suffering with HIV report nerve pain as the first symptom leading to diagnosis of the disease. There are frequent nerve tremors and spasms that occur in this disease.

Shingles

Shingles is the reactivation of the chickenpox virus in the body. A patient will experience a painful rash. The virus also has been found to attack the nerves in that area. Even after the resolution of the rash, the patient will continue to have nerve pain. Nerve pain can worsen as the disease progresses.

Types of Nerve Pain

Along with Sciatic Nerve Pain (SNP), pain is categorized as three major types. These types depend on the location the pain is felt in a human body. These three types of pain are as follows:

Somatic Nerve Pain

Somatic is basically a skin, muscle or tissue pain. The nerves that detect somatic pain are located deep in the skin tissues. Somatic pain can be easily treated as it is easy to isolate by the brain.

Symptoms may include inflammation, abnormal muscle twitching, fatigue, and weakness. Ibuprofen, Naprosyn and Tylenol are common names you will see on medications to treat somatic pain.

Visceral Nerve Pain

Visceral pain refers to a pain that arises from internal organs. It is difficult to locate as compared to somatic pain since the pain may be in the organs such as the kidney, stomach, intestines, bladder, etc.

The symptoms associated with it are nausea, fever, pain, and a malaise such as restlessness, depression, anxiety, or any general feeling of discomfort.

Treating visceral pain involves a wide variety of drugs which are heavier in composition than those used for somatic pain. This includes drugs such as opiates, anti-spasmodics, and anti-depressants.

Somatic pain and visceral pain may also be referred to as nociceptive pain by your doctor.

Neuropathic Nerve Pain

The third type of pain associated with SNP is neuropathic pain, which includes nerve damage.

This kind of pain is more chronic and complex than somatic and visceral pain. This is because nerve fibres are dysfunctional, damaged, or at times even dead.

Neuropathic pain may include nerve damage as well; these damaged nerves send the wrong signals to various pain centres in the body. However, this pain does not start abruptly. Symptoms may be intermittent in the beginning and then become chronic where it causes a constant burning. Patients may also feel immense pain at the slightest touch.

It is often believed that neuropathic pain is due to a problem in the peripheral nerves, like that which begins due to neuropathy caused by diabetes or stenosis. However, neuropathic pain can also be experienced with injuries that affect the brain or spinal cord.

Other causes of neuropathic pain may include alcoholism, amputation, chemotherapy, HIV/AIDS, and even certain spine surgeries. Conventional neuropathic treatment can be administered through massage therapies, meditation, acupuncture, and other physical therapies, while drugs such as Aleve and Motrin often help relieve the pain.

Somatic, visceral and neuropathic pain can either be acute or chronic. Acute pain can go away quickly and is comparatively easier to treat. Acute pain can also be the result of injury or infection. However, acute pain may develop into chronic pain if left untreated. Chronic pain is difficult to treat successfully and requires a different approach than what is currently offered.

Section 2

How to Treat Nerve Pain

Treating nerve pain can be tricky because the reason for the nerve pain is not always known. Unless the patient's nerve pain is due to a known medical condition, such as a severe disease (diabetes, cancer, or HIV), it is difficult to discover what is causing nerve pain.

The first step toward treatment is to identify the underlying cause, whether it's a deficiency of nutrients or an imbalance of hormones, a sleep disorder, some physical injury, or depression.

Finding the root cause of the problem is the most important part of treating nerve pain. Dealing with the symptoms and not the root cause is the conventional method that is widely used.

The following are treatments for mild nerve pain.

Applying Topical Ointments

Topical ointments are helpful to deal with immediate nerve pain symptoms. There are several creams, gels, and lotions that are readily available on the market as an instant remedy to treat nerve pain. In most cases, these topical ointments work in a few hours, treating the pain at its roots.

Taking Pain Killers and Anticonvulsants

Pain killers are the second option that you can use for the treatment of nerve pain. There are hundreds of pain killers, some can even be taken without a prescription to treat immediate nerve pain.

Anticonvulsants, though instantly effective, can be risky. If you are willing to use anticonvulsants for treatment of nerve pain, you must first visit your doctor and use only his prescribed drugs.

Eating Healthy

If your nerve pain is followed by weakness and a low blood pressure, it could mean that your body is not getting a good supply of essential nutrients. The most natural option for treating nerve pain is to start eating healthy immediately. Include in your diet vegetables, leafy greens, fruits, and nuts to regain the lost balance of nutrition.

Also, keep your body hydrated with 8-9 glasses of water each day.

Taking Vitamin Supplements

Vitamin supplements are another handy option that can work faster than eating healthy, because it gives all the power of essential nutrients in a tablet or tasty gummy.

Start taking multivitamin supplements on a regular basis to provide your body with the necessary nutrients. Other supplements that can help are alpha lipoic acid, omega fatty acids, and B vitamins. You must, however, opt for this option after consulting your healthcare professional.

Daily Working Out

Working out is the healthiest and second most natural option to deal with nerve pain. Develop a healthy lifestyle which includes walking, running, and exercise for 30 minutes a day. This can not only keep nerve pain at bay, but can also combat diabetes, cancer, and HIV which are the parent diseases of nerve pain.

Stretching and Relaxing

Stretch, relax, and meditate if your nerve pain is the result of anxiety and depression. This is the best remedy to defeat both depression and nerve pain single-handedly. Though it takes some time, it gives lasting results without stress on the body.

Regular Massage

Most of the time, nerve pain is caused by poor blood circulation. Sometimes the pain is because of the small amount of blood reaching the affected part of the body, while other times it is due to an excessive amount of blood flow.

Regular massage gives your body a steady and healthy blood flow, keeping all your organs, muscles, and tissues fully functional.

Try a hot oil massage for at least a week in the area where the pain occurs before trying other alternatives.

Chiropractic Care

Chiropractic is a great option to help with nerve pain. Nerve pain can result from nerve compression stemming from the spinal cord. An adjustment may be able to relieve the pressure allowing the nerve to heal as well as re-aligning the spinal segments.

Acupuncture

Acupuncture is a Chinese healing therapy in which needles are inserted into the affected part of the body. This method has gained some acceptance in the western world because of its effectiveness.

Acupuncture has been proven to be effective for the treatment of nerve pain in several research studies carried out worldwide. If you have a consistent nerve pain that isn't alleviated even after taking pain killers and applying ointments, you can try acupuncture. It has fewer risks or side-effects than other treatments.

Electrical Stimulation

Electrical stimulation is used independently and as part of surgery to treat nerve pain that is caused by milder levels of nerve damage. An electric impulse is used to stimulate neurological response and keep it from sensing pain messages sent by damaged nerves.

Section 3

How A Poor Diet Affects Your Happiness

Did you know a poor diet is the biggest cause of early death in the world? A study carried out in 2016 concluded the following:

- Unhealthy eating causes diabetes and heart disease, leading to an early death

- Blood pressure and smoking are the greatest risk factors for an early death

- 21% of global deaths were due to an excessive intake of sugary drinks and red meat

Source: Dailymail.co.uk

Based on this information, you can draw other conclusions as well. Eating healthy prolongs life, right?

However, the hullabaloo of daily life and tight work schedules doesn't support long-term healthy lifestyles. It keeps us so busy that we often do not have time for a glass of water.

Sometimes, we do realize we are missing out on the important things by focusing on work or other frivolous elements of life. Most of the time, however, we don't. We let unimportant things over shadow thoughts of living a healthy life.

But you know, just like time won't wait for you to succeed, life won't wait for you to eat properly. What would you do if your busy life has you on the run and you only have 15 minutes to eat? What would you choose?

Are you a fan of fast food and easy snacks? Are you addicted to frozen meals or having a cup of coffee as a meal? Is this an example of how you would eat? Because this is unhealthy eating.

You know what is better? Cooking veggies complimented with nuts, fruits, and a healthy amount of lean protein in your kitchen.

You knew that. So why is it that we know what to do, but we don't? The answer is that we are not looking forward to the future. We are not seeing what will happen to us until it is too late.

What is a Poor Diet?

A poor diet is high in calories, excessive salt, and saturated fats. It can also be one with not enough vitamins or minerals consumed by the body.

Excessive eating is the poorest type of diet. A healthy diet is one of balance. If you do not maintain an adequate proportion of vitamins, minerals, carbohydrates, and fats, you are not allowing your body to work the way it wants to.

A poor diet is also one that starves the body for a long time or one where you don't take your meals on a regular schedule. Your body is programmed to work on a schedule. When you deviate from that schedule things such as digestion and metabolism just will not work properly.

Our bodies have developed over time to adjust and create a state of balance. When we deprive our body of the nutrients it needs, it enters a state of adaptation. What that amounts to is a change in metabolic processes to deal with the situation. If you are skipping meals, you are training your body to be in a constant state of crisis. In the end, this means that critical processes are going to be altered.

Maybe you are eating and drinking healthily and on a proper schedule, but you weaken your diet with smoking and unhealthy drinking. Trust me, those poor habits make your healthy eating in vain.

Look at the pyramid below.

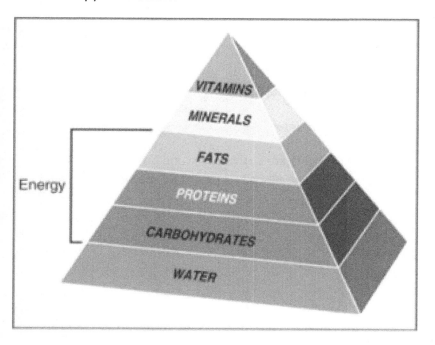

The pyramid arranges every nutrient in order of preference. Water is the foundation for life. Then carbohydrates, unsaturated fats, and proteins give you the energy to keep up with the pace of your life. Finally, minerals and vitamins make you strong, smart, and healthy in the long run.

Simply put, if any of the above nutrients are overprovided, underprovided, or irregularly provided to your body for a long period of time, you are making it hard for your body to work right.

Consequences of a Poor Diet

You must never neglect your dietary issues. People with a poor diet face innumerable health and weight problems which in the long run take shape as severe disease that can be fatal.

Let's have a look at what these problems can be so that you can stay aware of the consequences of a poor diet.

Short Term Consequences

Stress and Anxiety

Stress and anxiety are both a cause and product of a poor diet. They follow a poor diet and a poor diet follows them. It goes in a circle with no point of origin. But the good news is that it can end with a little concentration and effort invested in a special diet to counteract the effects of stress and anxiety.

Depression

Though depression is often due to a serious life trauma its effect increases when you have a poor diet. Also, getting over depression is harder when you are not eating healthy. Therefore, healthy eating keeps your happiness hormones stable.

Fatigue

A poor diet can make you feel tired and exhausted most of the time. You don't feel like working, going out, or even mating because your cells are not flush with essential nutrients.

If you are currently facing any of these issues, you are possibly lacking good nutrients in your body. Consult your nutritionist and seek a special dietary plan. A few supplements can give you amazing results in a few months while you add natural organic food into your diet.

Long Term Consequences

A poor diet can be worse in the long run as well. If the short-term consequences are not immediately addressed, it can expand and take shape as a serious and sometimes deadly disease.

Here are the greater risks posed by an unhealthy or poor diet.

Obesity

In the United States, 36.5% of adults and 17% of kids are obese according to a report by the Centres for Disease Control and Prevention. This rate is alarming.

Obesity is defined as an excess of adipose tissue. This problem continues to disturb health systems of the world today. Not only does obesity affect a person's weight but also the mortality, morbidity, and disability rate of a country.

How do you determine obesity?

If your body weight is 20% above the average and your Body Mass Index (BMI) is above 30, you are likely to be obese.

Obesity contributes to 30 of the most chronic diseases in medical history. They include cardiovascular disease, diabetes (type 1 and type 2), high blood pressure, gout, breathing problems, and cancer.

Cancer

Look at the following graph to understand the relationship of a poor diet with cancer.

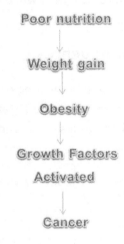

It shows that poor nutrition may lead to obesity if a person experiences a constant weight gain. However, the case may not always stay this simple. Being obese can cause several types of cancer, including cancers of the esophagus, thyroid, brain, breast (in postmenopausal women), liver, upper stomach, gall bladder, bowel, or colorectal. So, obesity can be fatal by leading to cancer.

Approximately 1 in 5 cancers in the U.S are associated with obesity according to the American Cancer Society. The question is how does obesity lead to cancer in your body?

Obesity brings extra fat. Fat cells activate growth hormones and other growth factors such as proteins. Hormones typically encourage cell proliferation. When you have a cancer cell that is exposed to hormones, the cell will grow and grow faster. This is typically why an oncologist will restrict anyone who has had breast cancer or prostate cancer from using any hormones, whether natural or synthetic.

Diabetes

A poor diet often causes type 1 and type 2 diabetes. When a person has poor nutrition, he is probably consuming unhealthy sugars, calories, and fats in sodas and other junk foods. This disturbs sugar levels greatly.

If sugar intake isn't controlled, diabetes takes root. Obese or over-weight people are reluctant to use more insulin to control blood sugar levels. Hence, they are more exposed to fatal diseases like diabetes. Due to a poor diet and unhealthy eating habits, childhood diabetes has become very common across the globe.

Cardiovascular Disease

When we talk about poor nutrition and obesity, cardiovascular disease is the first thing that clicks in our minds.

Around 70% of adults in America are at a risk of heart attack, atherosclerosis and high blood pressure. Previously it was thought that fats were inert and did not have an impact on your body. However, more recently scientists have researched that fat impacts your metabolism and how your body functions. Fat disturbs metabolism by affecting lipid levels (HDL and LDL), blood pressure and the use of insulin.

Changes in blood pressure levels (normal to high) and an abnormal lipid profile cause increased exposure to heart disease. Fat droplets often get stuck in arteries, decreasing the surface area of the artery. This causes serious concerns such as atherosclerosis and angina.

Osteoporosis

Osteoporosis is caused by inadequate reserves of calcium and vitamin D in the body.

The symptoms involve immense back pain, frequent fractures, a loss in height and a stooped posture. This occurs when bones lose their density due to an extreme deficiency of calcium and phosphate.

Calcium and vitamin D supplements in combination with a daily intake of fortified milk and yogurt can ease the situation in early stages. However, in the late phase of life it is likely to be a long-term issue.

Anaemia

One of the most common disorders caused by poor nutrition is anaemia. It is when your body lacks the most basic yet powerful mineral: iron.

When iron is deficient, your body is unable to make haemoglobin, which carries the oxygen in red blood cells essential for tissues and muscles to function properly. Anaemia may result in fatigue, headache, irregular heartbeat, pale skin and other serious conditions.

To prevent or treat anaemia, one must eat foods rich in iron such as apples, cranberries, cherries or beef and poultry products. One may also take vitamin B-12 and iron supplements after consulting a nutritionist.

Rickets

Rickets is a disease which results from a serious deficiency of vitamin D, and affects the development of bones in children. Rickets results in major problems associated with the health of a growing child, increasing the chances of fracture, bone softening, muscle pain, and other deformities.

Scurvy

Scurvy is a painful disease caused by the deficiency of vitamin C. Patients with scurvy may face severe anaemia, ulceration of the gums, and other tooth problems such as loss of teeth in a short time span.

Now, do you think you can lead a happy life when you are suffering one disease or another? No. Life is happy only when it is healthy; and it is healthy with a balanced and nutritional diet.

Steps for Improving your Diet

Here is how you can improve your diet with a little effort.

Set a Meal Planner

The first step to a healthy diet is to plan. You are not a computer and so don't expect to remember all that you need to include or exclude from your diet. Write it down. Make a quick search of the healthiest veggies, fruits, nuts, and grains and how to cook them in a meal.

Set your schedule with particular meals. For example, take Monday:

Breakfast. Fruit salad with a glass of water

Lunch: Spinach rolls with an orange or papaya

Dinner: Fish with a vegetable salad

This way, you will have an organized schedule for the week. Also, a chart can help you plan your grocery shopping accordingly.

Eat on Time

A proper schedule is as important as eating healthy. If you are taking meals at odd hours and without any connection with a previous meal time, it is futile. Your body has an internal clock when it comes to some essential functions. Maintaining a regular eating schedule makes it easier for your body to function effectively.

Make a time chart for your meals. If you have your breakfast at 8 in the morning, try to have it at 8 regularly. The same goes for lunch and dinner, or even if you take split meals.

Keep Yourself Hydrated

Drinking plenty of water is necessary. Water deficiency can damage your organs and decrease their function. Drink 8-9 glasses a day.

Say No to Sugary Sweets

No matter how finicky your sweet tooth is, keep it under control. Eliminate sugary drinks, desserts, and candies in your diet. Look for healthy sweet alternatives such as dark chocolate, dates, and fruits.

Take Vitamin Supplements

In the end, it's good to talk to your nutritionist about ways to improve your diet. If he/she suggests, add supplements that would support the required amount of vitamins in your body. Vitamins improve immunity and trigger organ functionality.

Section 4

What is wrong with the food we eat?

As explained earlier, a poor diet is an unbalanced diet. When you feel lethargic and tired all the time there is certainly something fishy with your diet.

The question is, what actually is wrong with the food you eat? You think by going to a high-end restaurant or a renowned fast food chain they'll serve you freshly prepared food which is made under hygienic conditions, so there's nothing wrong with it. But there is.

The point is, those prepared meals are French fries and nuggets as appetizers, cheese burgers and pizzas as main courses, and a soda for dessert. Does this sound familiar? All these meals sound mesmerizing and delightful to the taste buds but they come loaded with an abundance of calories, saturated fats, and excessive sugars, making them poor choices.

It's high time you realize that even when you get a sub sandwich and load it with many fresh veggies, making you think it is healthy, there are other things that can change it from healthy to unhealthy.

Let's learn what these other things are.

Cheese

Those cheesiest of burgers, pizzas, cream cheese pastas, parmesan-coated breads, and other divine pleasures of cheese are just heaven on Earth, aren't they? Yes, they certainly are.

Even though cheese has all the dietary elements of milk, being a dairy product, and it is a good source of vitamins A and D, too much cheese can bring detrimental effects to your body.

So, cheese always has the potential to turn your diet options to an unhealthy or poor choice.

Cheese can be a source of fat and cholesterol and this can cause problems such as weight gain or obesity and can even lead to cardiovascular diseases in extreme cases.

Some types of cheese contain high levels of sodium that may cause high blood pressure. Therefore, make sure you keep cheese on the side of a balanced diet.

Salt

Most recipes suggest you 'add salt to taste' when it comes to the amount of salt in your food. You need a sufficient level of salt in your diet to maintain a normal blood pressure but, as too much of anything is harmful, excessive salt can also cause problems.

The Dietary Guidelines for Americans in 2010 suggests the daily intake of salt shall be no more than 2300 milligrams, which amounts to one teaspoon.

For patients with high blood pressure, diabetes and other kidney and cardiovascular problems, the recommended daily intake is no more than 1500 milligrams of salt per day.

Excessive salt in a diet increases our vulnerability to diseases such as high blood pressure, resulting in strokes and other cardio problems, kidney stones, dementia and much more.

Junk Food

Foods with high levels of calories, sugars, and fats are junk foods. They have no health benefits, being low in vitamins, minerals, fibre, and proteins that are the key nutrients to an essential diet.

The typical diet we see people eat have things like burgers, pizzas, and French fries. These are foods that have been given to us as children. We now see them as a part of our lives. Science and research has shown that if we continue to eat out of convenience, there are devastating consequences.

Change your eating habits not only for you, but to show your children what healthy eating should be. Give them a chance at a better and healthier life.

Sauces

This is an underestimated and overlooked sphere that can damage the diet. There is much talk about the harm of eating fatty burgers and cheesy pizzas but very little light is shed on what makes these burgers and pizzas such a darling to the taste buds. It is the sauces: ketchups, barbeque sauce, mustard sauce, soy sauce, chilli sauce, mayonnaise, etc.

It is easy to cut burgers from a diet and say, "I have made a good choice." But you have not if you are still consuming the sauces. People cook vegetables and dip them in sauces. What is left of the good effect of a vegetable?

Sauces have artificial colours, flavours, fats, and other ingredients that are a slow poison to your body. Never be duped by the nutrition label on the bottle of a sauce. It always comes with a lot of dangerous health risks.

To stay healthy, keep these away from your diet and try to familiarize your taste buds with more natural food options.

Breads and Buns

In today's society, lunch for most people involves some kind of bread. Society has made us associate lunch with two pieces of bread and meat as what you should eat.

Breads and buns are made with flour and that's it. No vitamins, no minerals, no fibre, and therefore no nutrition. They have no value in a healthy diet. And do not think adding some veggies to a bun can make it healthy. No, never substitute a bread or a bun for organic wholegrain.

There are so many great options out their now for breads that are truly good for you. Look in your grocery stores for breads that contain seeds and protein as part of the bread.

Pre-packaged Juices

Pre-packaged juices are just another farce. All those ads and banners keep telling you that you can only get healthy when you drink a can of juice every morning. But what they hide is that their juice is processed with a lot of additives, preservatives, and harmful sugars that void the healthy content of a fruit.

If you must, then go only for the juice you extract yourself in a juicer. Only then are you sure it is 100% fresh and natural.

At this point, you might be thinking everything you eat today is leading you down the wrong path. Don't worry, there is always time to change.

It just takes dedication and being honest with yourself. Cut down the bad and replace it with what's good. We will discuss healthy food options in the later sections.

Section 5

What is the impact of the food we eat?

From early school days, we are taught about following a *balanced diet* to lead a healthy life. Some are prescribed a different diet depending on their health. For instance, a diabetic is not allowed to have sugar and a patient with high blood pressure is advised to limit salt. This differs from person to person according to their medical condition.

Every time we scroll through our newsfeeds, we see loads of pictures of foods and beverages and we keep hitting *like*. Our social media newsfeeds certainly show that we are obsessed with food, no matter what kind, be it traditional or contemporary. All we want to try are those mesmerizing flavours and mouth-watering spices from all over the globe.

Despite the drool and hype we have created for unique flavours and exquisite cuisines, every food has its advantages and disadvantages. Canned food, organic food, preservatives, artificial flavours and other such things can impact your diet. However, it would be extremely beneficial to know how certain foods specifically can bring positive and negative impacts on your diet. Time to go a bit more in depth! Following are the foods and their impact.

Organic versus Pre-made

In today's world, nothing is 100% pure and organic. The increasing popularity of junk food is leading to obesity which further drains a person's health. The food we eat plays a huge factor in biological dysfunction, in part because our diets lack the necessary balance of nutrients.

Artificial sweeteners and preservatives have been known to cause fibromyalgia and seizures. To heal your body, you must remove all the toxic foreign substances from your diet: artificial sweeteners, preservatives, fake dyes, and anything that has chemicals in it and is not directly from the land.

Supermarkets are full of conveniently packaged foods that appeal to our taste buds but compromise our nutrition. Most of these foods' natural nutrients are removed in the refining process.

Eat all natural; no mixtures. Homemade is the best!

Plant vegetables and fruits in your garden instead of purchasing them from the supermarket because you don't know if they're as pure and fresh as the store promises them to be.

Fast food, loved by many people, has its side effects: extra calories, insulin resistance, high blood pressure, bloating and puffiness, shortness of breath, depression, dental disease, weight problems, high cholesterol, headaches and acne.

Fat

Fat is not all bad and going on a crash diet or low-fat diet is not all good for your anatomy. The body requires some fat to stay fit. Fat provides insulation for the organs, transports fat-soluble vitamins (A, D, E, K), provides materials critical to the integrity of cellular membranes, lubricates mucous membranes and skin, provides materials used to make hormones, helps the body utilize glucose more effectively, contributes to healthy joints, promotes efficient gut health, facilitates immune system function and, depending on the type of fat, can increase or decrease inflammation. Enjoy beneficial fats. Get the majority of your fats from plants and fish, and minimize your intake of saturated animal fats.

Raw Food

Cooking or heating food makes them lose half of their nutritional value, including vitamins and protein. Having raw food is healthier for the body.

Vitamin C strengthens the immune system, eases nerve pain, repairs damaged nerves, lowers the risk of developing autoimmune diseases, slows the aging process, and increases metabolism. If you cook food rich in vitamin C, you are denaturing the food, thereby removing what your body needs.

An apple a day keeps the doctor away. Why?

Apples are a rich source of a variety of phytonutrients. Epidemiological studies have linked the consumption of apples with a reduced risk of cardiovascular disease, asthma, diabetes, and some cancers. Apples have been found to have very strong anti-oxidant activity, inhibit cancer cell proliferation, and decrease lipid oxidation and lower cholesterol. (Nutrition Journal, 2004).

Water

Most essential – water. Water is very important to nerve health! Water intake is mandatory. Your body is composed of 60% water. Drinking water helps maintain the balance of body fluids. The functions of these bodily fluids include digestion, absorption, circulation, creation of saliva, transportation of nutrients and maintenance of the body's temperature.

Meat

Go back to your friend's Instagram or just your newsfeed and notice what most of the people are putting up in their food pictures. You will notice that the food items pictured are mostly those of meat! It's a common trend and easy to notice. All you see will be meaty pizzas, sizzling beef steaks, tempting pastas with meat sauce, plus-sized beef burgers and other such meaty-licious items that all meat lovers drool over. However, meat has its own positive and negative impacts.

Meat, if processed well, has various nutrients. Approximately 3.5 ounces of raw ground beef contains a bulk of healthy nutrients such as B12, B3, B6, iron, zinc, selenium and several more vitamins as well. So, if you are one of those people who avoids meat, you must stop doing this since meat brings a lot of benefits to your body that are just as good as cuisines that do not contain meat. But as we have mentioned earlier, remember that too much of anything can be bad for you.

Meat has several drawbacks as well that can ruin your health. Let's have a look at these hazards.

- Excessive meat hardens blood vessels. A compound of meat called *carnitine* causes atherosclerosis and clogging of the arteries (source: Nature Medicine Journal).

- Your meat might be PINK SLIME. Preserved and canned meat can often be something called "lean finely textured beef," a processed meat that is treated with ammonia gas to kill bacteria. However, as per several research studies, this ammonia gas exposes the meat to many more pathogens which may grow further in your kitchen or refrigerator (source: Medical University South Carolina). This makes pink slime seriously unhealthy!

- Those breaded filets that you get might be *glued* together scraps. Transglutaminase is a meat glue that is made from a fermentation of bacteria. It is generally regarded as safe but it increases the risk of contamination, causing an unhealthy impact on your body if contamination does occur.

- You may be exposed to E-coli. Cattle present a major threat for E-coli, as per the CDC. This bacterium can make you extremely sick, causing dehydration, abdominal cramps, and kidney failure.

In this part, we discussed the impact of food items; meat specifically. Let's have a look at some more food items below to understand how they can bring a positive and negative impact on your diet.

Oil and Butter

These two items are commonly used in almost every food preparation across the globe and are available in every super-market with a wide variety of brands. Oil and butter are, in fact, two special ingredients in the traditional Asian foods that we eat and they have both a positive and negative impact.

- Oil and butter are a great source of energy which is required by the body to perform its functions.

- Certain butter oils are also rich in arachidonic acid (AA) which is an omega-6 fatty acid.

- Real butter has an extremely rich vitamin content and anti-oxidants that prevent free radical damage.

- Despite its benefits, we can also see certain negatives that it brings to food when added in excessive amounts, such as with foods like French fries, buttered buns/rolls and other fatty foods like cheese, mayonnaise, and salad dressings. They increase the amount of high density lipids in our body, add excessive fat and may result in obesity and cardiovascular disease in the long-term.

Hence, the impact of the food we eat can be both positive and negative. We need to set priorities toward each food and the appropriate portion size to maintain a balanced diet.

Section 6

How Pharmaceutical Drugs Affect People with a Poor Diet

Mind over matter. How many weight loss pills do you come across and believe that by taking them, without changing your eating habits, it will lead you to the ideal figure? Everything comes with a price. A healthy, clean diet would be helpful to lose those extra pounds rather than to depend on medication while you keep stuffing your mouth with anything you please.

Anti-depressant pills are guaranteed to make you feel better although all they do is mask the symptoms. There will come a point when the medication stops working. Doctors would typically increase the dosage or change to a stronger medication but with every medication there is always a side effect. If you are following a poor diet, these medications are going to affect your organs and systems in a negative way.

One must have a good *nutritional* intake to fight any condition, be it physical or mental. For depression, you are advised to eat fatty fish (anchovy, mackerel, salmon, sardines, shad, and tuna), flaxseed, canola and soybean oils, nuts (especially walnuts), and dark green leafy vegetables. These foods provide the nutrients the body needs to fight off inflammation in the brain, which leads to depression.

Taking medicine on an empty stomach is not advised, because when your body has no energy it cannot absorb the dosage of medicine, leading to a worsening of your condition. Augmentin is usually prescribed for many different infections caused by bacteria, such as sinusitis, pneumonia, ear infections, bronchitis, urinary tract infections, infections of the skin, and fever. Although it is there to help you feel better it has its side effects too: mild diarrhea, gas, stomach pain, nausea or vomiting, headache, skin rash or itching, white patches in your mouth or throat, or vaginal yeast infection (itching or discharge).

For a wound, it is very common in the eastern world to treat with turmeric and milk. Turmeric has been used as a spice in Indian recipes and as an Ayurvedic medicine for thousands of years. Turmeric offers many health benefits since it has anti-inflammatory and anti-oxidant properties. It is used to relieve swelling and pain due to headaches and wounds and is called a 'natural aspirin' in Ayurvedic medicine. It also possesses anti-bacterial properties and when applied to small cuts and wounds, it can stem blood flow by aiding with clotting, prevent infections and heal wounds. Combined with milk, turmeric is used as a drink, lotion or even a face mask.

This all-natural cure for a variety of ailments is safe to use. Milk, we all know, strengthens bones. Combined with turmeric it provides additional benefits to bone health. This remedy has no side effects, unlike pharmaceuticals which don't really suit every situation.

For pain, there are medications like ibuprofen or acetaminophen. They surely come with benefits but there are always side effects. These side effects become even more potent if you are in poor health. Some of the commonly reported side effects of ibuprofen include: haemorrhage, vomiting, anaemia, decreased haemoglobin, eosinophilia, and hypertension. Other side effects include: upper gastrointestinal haemorrhage, upper gastrointestinal tract ulcer, dizziness, and dyspepsia. See below for a comprehensive list of adverse effects. You can only imagine if you already had these problems and you were on medication, that the side effects would be GREATER!

As per a study conducted by the Geriatric Medicine Departments of England, Wales and Scotland, approximately 15.3% of patients experienced adverse effects of pharmaceutical drugs. They also found out that hypotensive drugs, anti-Parkinsonian drugs and psychotropic drugs carried a high risk of adverse effects on human health. Moreover, people with a poor diet have a weak immune system and their metabolism isn't healthy enough to remove toxins which are created by the break-down of drugs in the body. Hence, they are more exposed to adverse effects of pharmaceutical drugs.

The following is a list of adverse effects that may be due to a pharmaceutical drug.

- Excessive sweating

- Abnormal blood pressure

- Gastro-intestinal problems such as ulcers in extreme cases

- Skin allergies or rash

- Vertigo and nausea

- Increased pain, rather than decreased pain

- Diarrhea

- Drowsiness

If you experience any such side effects after taking a pharmaceutical drug, you must immediately consult a doctor. Let's learn more about the adverse effects of some commonly used pharmaceutical drugs that are found in almost every house, at least periodically.

- Paracetamol. You must have had Panadol or Calpol! Paracetamol, also known as acetaminophen (biological name), is a pharmaceutical drug used to relieve pain and fever. Whether it is a back breaking pain, a terrible headache or a chill-and-aches kind of fever, most people would first pop an acetaminophen. Here are some side effects: nausea, vomiting, loss of appetite, or severe stomach pain. Additionally, light headiness, sweating, fatigue, or weakness.

- Amoxicillin. One of the most commonly used pharmaceutical drugs, amoxicillin also causes certain side effects such as abdominal or stomach cramps, black tarry stools, tooth problems, blood in urine, nose bleeds, severe chest pain, heavier menstrual periods, bloating, abnormal heart beat, loss of appetite and inflammation of joints, etc.

When it comes to a poor diet, you're putting your body more at risk to the side effects of pharmaceutical drugs. You may be amazed to know that a poor diet and such side-effects have a relationship that is directly connected. Imagine being obese because of a poor diet and you start taking weight reduction drugs. Eventually these weight reduction drugs may cause various side effects! Let's consider a few weight-reduction drugs and know their adverse effects.

- Xenical, also known as Orlistat, is a gastrointestinal lipase inhibitor that is one of the most widely used drugs for weight loss. It aids weight loss by restricting the digestion and absorption of fat in the body by inhibiting the enzyme lipase. This is certainly a complex process as lipase does work as a common part of our digestive system. It can bring various side effects such as flatulence, urgent bowel movements (decreasing control over bowel function), nausea, vomiting, rectal pain, loss of appetite, skin allergies, jaundice, dark urine, tooth decay and much more.

- Lorcaserin, currently known as Belviq, was developed by Arena Pharmaceuticals and acts as an anorectic or dietary suppressant. It was approved in year 2012 to be used as a drug to treat obesity. However, even though it is approved, certain adverse effects are associated with it although they aren't as serious as naltrexone. The side effects of lorcaserin are comprised of headaches, dizziness, drowsiness, fatigue, dry mouth, constant cough and back pain.

Pharmaceutical drugs, whether associated with a poor diet or not, always cause adverse effect on the human body. You should notice in the first few doses if you are experiencing any kind of side effect. If so, then immediately contact your doctor and stop taking such pharmaceutical drugs. Instead, move toward naturally made things such as herbs and many fruit and vegetable juices which help cure your problems and can help cleanse your blood by flushing away the toxins.

Section 7

The Ramifications of Poor Nutrition and Consuming Pain Killers

In the present world, where various developments have been made in the fields of health and medicine, the use/abuse of painkillers and the increasing trends of eating out/unhealthy eating have become a growing concern for doctors and nutritionists across the globe.

Let's discuss some ramifications associated with poor nutrition and excessive use and abuse of pain killers.

Pain Killers

Having a little headache? Having a little back pain? All you need are a few painkillers that you can go grab from the cupboard or drawer. However, this SHOULD NOT be the case.

About 76,000 American NSAID users are hospitalized each year due to ulcers and other side effects caused by prescription pain killers, and about 7,600 of those users die from the ulcers caused by these painkillers. But despite the various side effects, we continue to use pain killers excessively even when we can easily manage the situation without them.

These prescription pain killers have been causing thousands of deaths along with various other medical concerns on a global scale. Let's review the common risks associated with painkillers.

- ***Over dose in children***
  One of the most common problems for children associated
  with painkillers is over dosing. If children are given two
  times the normal dose, they will face an over dose which
  can cause liver damage and even be fatal.

- ***Some painkillers may have cancer causing toxins***
  Benadryl, Tylenol, Motrin and Sudafed, if taken excessively,
  may cause cancer since they do have cancer causing toxins.
  These toxins or compounds are lactose, mannitol, sorbitol,
  sucrose, inositol, FD&C YELLOW No. 3 & 40 and FD&C Blue
  No. 1 & 2.

- ***Liver and kidney damage***
  The American Medical Association (AMA) states that each
  year around 50,000 people go to the emergency room for
  kidney and liver damage due to the side effects of
  painkillers.

- ***Increased pain rather than decreased pain***
  Motrin can increase your headache rather than decreasing
  it. The side effects of Motrin include diarrhea, dizziness and
  even headache. Which means it may increase rather than
  stabilize your pain!

Poor Nutrition

Poor nutrition may sound simple, but it's not. It's complex
because it affects the entire mechanism of your body, be it a
cell, organ or a nerve. Your body requires many nutrients in a
balanced diet and poor nutrition may result when one of the
essential nutrients is missing for a prolonged period. Each
nutrient has its vital role in your body and fulfilment of these
roles lets your body function properly.

For example, you need a sufficient amount of carbohydrates in your diet to acquire energy. Your body starts to break down stored fats if there are insufficient carbohydrates. A breakdown of these fats produces lactic acid that, in excess, isn't very good for your health. Similarly, nutrients like fibre also play a vital role; they help you avoid constipation and maintain a healthy digestive system. Water is also considered a nutrient and is extremely essential for chemical reactions happening in every cell of your body. Hence, staying hydrated is also a part of proper nutrition.

Other nutrients such as proteins are vital for cell growth and development. Every nutrient plays a distinct role and you must have specific proportions of each nutrient in your diet. Sticking to a diet which is only protein or only carb is never a good idea! Visit a dietician soon if you think that your diet is poor in nutrition to avoid all the consequences associated with it.

Despite all the ramifications we know are associated with pain killers and poor nutrition, we are still unable to escape them. We are surrounded by them and recent generations have become a victim of our unhealthy lifestyles. We must remember that *health is wealth.* For that reason, we must try to avoid excessive and unnecessary use of pain killers and must be health conscious to avoid the myriad of problems that are associated with poor nutrition or malnutrition.

Along with the various side effects of pain killers and poor diet that we discussed earlier in this section, let's shed more light on this important and long neglected issue.

First, let's talk a bit more about pain killers.

When you feel drained due to immense pain in your back, neck or muscles, you would obviously move toward a strong painkiller that immediately remedies the pain. Hence, it would be good to know what effect pain killers have on your body.

Opioids have a morphine-like effect on the body by producing opioid receptors to relieve pain. They are known as the most powerful pain killers of all times and are legally available, but strictly by prescription. Examples include some renowned and extensively used pain killers such as oxycodone (OxyContin), hydrocodone (Vicodin), codeine, morphine and fentanyl.

However, there are also a weaker type of these opioids, such as codeine and dihydrocodeine. Side effects of these opioids are major. Let's have a look at them below.

- **Addiction.** People can get hooked on these pain killers, wanting them even when their need isn't necessary.
- **Breathing problems**. Respiratory depression is a major drawback of opioids. This is due to the way these painkillers operate on respiratory centres in the brain.
- **Slow response and confusion**. Opioids can cause cognitive changes due to the way these painkillers work on the central nervous system (CNS). "You feel less sharp, you think a little bit slower, it kind of slows your coordination," says Dr. Chou (health.com).
- **Constipation**. Painkillers work on pain receptors that also affect the gut. Researchers believe that almost all drugs can affect the gut, causing constipation.
- **Drowsiness**. Approximately 20 to 60% of patients see an increase in the amount of time they sleep when taking opioid painkillers.

- **Allergic reaction.** Around 2 to 10% of people who take opioids experience serious allergic reactions.
- **Nausea.** Around 25% of patients experience severe nausea after they start taking opioids. The nausea tends to fade away after time as you get used to the opioids.
- **Sexual side effects**. Using opioids for chronic pain may affect your sex life. Researchers are still discussing how opioids cause changes in sexual hormones but it has been proven that both male and female opioid users experience difficulty in achieving orgasm. Males often experience erectile dysfunction because opioids lower the levels of the male sex hormone testosterone.

These are just some of the ramifications caused by commonly used opioids. Now it would be beneficial to know more about a poor diet. Earlier in this section, we discussed the consequences of a poor diet. Now let's shed some further light on how a poor diet can be fixed and made better, rather than letting the situation worsen. Following is a table of certain effects discussed earlier and details about how it can be fixed.

RESULTS OF A POOR DIET	HOW IT CAN BE IMPROVED?
WEIGHT GAIN	Weight gain certainly sounds simple, but it has a lot of things related to it. The problems usually start with being over-weight. If you find out that your Body Mass Index is in the range of 25 to 30, cut down on excessive caloric intake and immediately begin working out in some way. Engage in activities such as walking, biking, swimming, jogging or indulge in other sports activities that interest you.
OBESITY	This is one of the worst consequences of a

	poor diet! Obesity, as stated earlier, can lead to various diseases. Therefore, it needs to be fixed as soon as possible. If you find that your Body Mass Index is 30 or higher, you must be aware that you are classified as obese. Follow a strict diet, even stricter than the one you would follow for weight gain discussed above. Avoid all excessive calories and do not skip your work-out routine. Since the diet should be proper, make sure you go to a nutritionist rather than try and tackle the issue by yourself. Make simple changes at first, such as using stairs rather than elevators, using whole grain bread instead of white bread, and walking rather than using a car.
NUTRIENT DEFICIENCY	Doctors often suggest that you have blood tests and other vitamin/nutrient tests about every six months to know if everything is normal. If you do not check on this regularly, long term deficiencies of nutrients such as calcium, vitamin D, iron, etc. may cause you to suffer great setbacks. Therefore, keep a check on your health first and foremost. Second, if you are deficient in any nutrient or if you feel any symptoms explained elsewhere in this book, immediately visit a doctor. The doctor may prescribe the use of supplements and suggest other natural food items for you to consume.

So far, we know a great deal about the ramifications of a poor diet and over use of painkillers. To avoid these consequences, maintain a balance of your activities and what you eat. Love yourself enough to avoid these outcomes, or fix them once identified, rather than just finding a way to live with them.

Section 8

Nerve pain and nerve damage have become a growing concern in this era. There is widespread suffering and people have been spending loads of money on pharmaceutical drugs and strong painkillers to treat nerve pain and nerve damage. Nerve pain and nerve damage can vary from person to person, as can its causes. It might stem from hereditary factors, a metabolic disorder, inflammation, diabetes, aging or any number of other factors. Doctors across the globe use several distinguished methods to treat nerve pain and nerve damage. Some use over-the-counter painkillers or pharmaceutical drugs like morphine or warren, while others may suggest therapy, meditation and Ayurveda herbs that help to cure nerve pain and nerve damage.

Let's first examine some of the foods that you shall be using to cure these disorders.

20 Miraculous Foods That Can Reverse Nerve Damage and Reduce Pain

Green Juicing

Green juicing is very important as it stops the cycle of chronic inflammation and gets inflamed nerves back in shape. Green juices are made with fruits and vegetables filled with antioxidants, phytochemicals, minerals and vitamins. Juicing is not any healthier than eating whole fruits and vegetables. The resulting liquid contains most of the vitamins, minerals and plant chemicals (phytonutrients) found in the whole fruit. Juicing cucumbers, celery, kale, parsley, spinach, broccoli, and any other greens gets you back on track. Green juicing helps clean toxins from body that might be causing nerve pain.

Ginger

Ginger is great for nerve pain. Gingerol is the main bioactive compound in ginger, responsible for much of its medicinal properties. It has powerful anti-inflammatory and antioxidant effects. It helps to get rid of the inflammation in all of the body's nerves. It's used as a traditional stomach soother, easing seasickness and nausea, and is believed to work by breaking up intestinal gas and possibly blocking a receptor in the gut that induces vomiting. As a natural alternative to aspirin and anti-inflammatory medicine, it can offer relief from migraines, arthritis pain, and muscle aches.

Cherry

Cherries are considered one of the best fruits to cleanse the body and release toxins. "They block inflammation and they inhibit pain enzymes, just like aspirin, naproxen, and other nonsteroidal anti-inflammatories," says Muraleedharan Nair, PhD, a natural products chemist at Michigan State University's College of Agricultural and Natural Resources.

Cherries contain powerful antioxidants like anthocyanin and cyanide. These have many benefits such as reducing belly fat, supporting healthy sleep, lowering the risk of stroke, and providing cancer preventive compounds and arthritis pain relief.

Cranberry

Cranberry juice helps prevent ulcers, thanks to its ability to block *H. pylori* from adhering to the stomach lining. Many of these phytonutrients offer antioxidant, anti-inflammatory and anti-cancer health benefits. Cranberries are a very good source of vitamin C, dietary fibre, and manganese, as well as a good source of vitamin E, vitamin K, copper and pantothenic acid.

Fish

Salmon, herring, and sardines help relieve back pain, as they are low in mercury and high in omega-3 fatty acids. These fish are also a good source of vitamin D and zinc.

Yogurt

Yogurt comes from milk, and everyone is aware of the benefits of milk. Yogurt gives a dose of animal protein (about 9 grams per 6-ounce serving), plus several other nutrients found in dairy foods like calcium, vitamin B-2, B-12, potassium, and magnesium. There's evidence that some strains of probiotics can help boost the immune system and promote a healthy digestive tract. Greek yogurt is typically the best choice.

Peppermint

There are many positive aspects to eating mint. Mint has one of the highest antioxidant levels of any food. Mint is good for stomach aches, bad breath, diarrhea, kidney stones, gallstones, headache, backache, neck pain, and altitude sickness.

Flaxseed

Apart from the herbs used to treat nerve pain, flaxseeds have been a blessing over the centuries in treating nerve damage. Flaxseeds contain omega-3, fibre, protein, vitamin B1, manganese, magnesium, phosphorus, vitamin B6, iron and selenium. Not only does flaxseed help in curing nerve damage but it is often used for treating cancer, menopausal symptoms, digestive problems, weight loss and to detoxify the blood. Arnica oils and creams are also widely available these days and they are being prescribed by homeopathic doctors to treat sprains, bruises and muscle/nerve pain.

Damiana

Damiana is a Mexican shrub. It does wonders for nerve pain caused by exercising too hard or by trauma to a specific body area. Damiana is also quite popular for its *magical* properties, including enhancing one`s sexual ability.

Peppermint and ginger

A diabetic patient at times endures sugar level fluctuations. When the blood sugar is down, a diabetic is prescribed to eat something sweet; glucose, juice, anything which is sugary. But when the sugar is high then what does one do? Mint and ginger are two foods which are good in healing nerve damage. Making a combo of these two, a few pieces of mint and a tiny slice of raw ginger, is good enough to bring that high sugar back to normal.

Water

Water is a necessity for survival. Water is the main ingredient in the body. Every cell in your body, and every function of those cells, is dependent on water. Staying hydrated has many beneficial attributes, like keeping your skin healthy. Lowering your body temperature is a direct result of staying hydrated as you exercise. Water is essential for the proper circulation of nutrients in the body and serves as the body's transportation system. When one is dehydrated things just can't get around well in your body.

Edamame

Edamame is a preparation of immature soybeans in the pod. When it comes to culinary fixes for pain, edamame is a tool for sore muscles. It has a high protein content and fewer calories, which make it an ideal snack for weight conscious people. The benefits of edamame include helping to keep a healthy digestive system as it is a good source of fibre which facilitates digestion.

Peppers

An ingredient in some peppers called capsaicin yields pain-fighting benefits by stimulating nerve endings and depleting a chemical that relays pain signals. The highest amount of vitamin C in a bell pepper is concentrated in the red variety. The capsaicin in bell peppers has multiple health benefits. Red bell peppers contain several phytochemicals and carotenoids, particularly beta-carotene, which provide anti-oxidant and anti-inflammatory benefits.

Omega-3 fish oil

Omega-3 fish oil contains both docosahexaenoic acid (DHA) and eicosapentaenoic acid (EPA). Omega-3 fatty acids are essential nutrients that are important in preventing and managing heart disease. They will help to sooth away inflammation and start the healing process. Also, the latest findings show that omega-3 fish oil helps in lowering blood pressure.

Skullcap

Skullcap is a powerful medicinal herb which helps to strengthen the nervous system and bring relief to agitated nerves that need attention.

Lobelia

Lobelia is a genus of flowering plants comprised of 415 species. It is another herb that helps to soothe, relax, and alleviate tension caused by contracted muscles which can put pressure on nerves.

Black Cohosh

Black cohosh helps to soothe and regenerate irritated nerves and get the body moving in the right direction for healing. It has been used by Native Americans for more than two hundred years, after they discovered the root of the plant helped relieve menstrual cramps and symptoms of menopause. It is still used for menopausal symptoms such as hot flashes/flushes, irritability, mood swings and sleep disturbances.

Antioxidants

An antioxidant is a molecule that inhibits the oxidation of other molecules. Oxidation is a chemical reaction that can produce free radicals, leading to chain reactions that may damage cells. Antioxidants such as thiols or ascorbic acid (vitamin C) terminate these chain reactions. Acai berry, camu camu fruit, grape seed extract, and avocado seed extract are great antioxidants.

Turmeric

Turmeric is one of the best herbs for pain. It stops the pain process and helps you to feel like new again.

Bitters

Bitters are traditionally an alcoholic preparation flavoured with botanical matter, such that the end result is characterized by a bitter, sour, or bittersweet flavour. Bitters help curb sugar cravings, soothe gas and bloating, calm upset stomachs and nausea, increase absorption of fat soluble vitamins (A, D, E, K), help maintain healthy blood sugar levels, balance the appetite and relieve occasional heartburn, digestive enzymes, bile & HCL production.

Herbs That Can Reverse Nerve Damage and Reduce Pain

Even though doctors usually use medical drugs to treat their patients with nerve damage and nerve pain, herbs are also used to a major extent in many cultures. Herbs heal wounds by promoting cell growth and repair. They also lower inflammation, help relax and soothe jangled nerves, lower stress, and help in the healing process of nerves. Herbs like vervain, wild lettuce, valerian, cramp bark, and St. John's wort are good for healing. We'll now take an in-depth review of the herbs that can be used to treat these disorders.

Ginseng

One of the best herbs used to treat nerve pain is ginseng, which is commonly found in North America and eastern Asia (mostly northeast China, Korea, Bhutan) but now countries across the globe are importing it as well. For centuries, ginseng has been used in traditional medicines and modern research has shown that it is great for neuron and nerve health. It helps improve memory, cures nerve pain, reduces the symptoms of menopause and reduces fatigue.

Kava-kava

Another herb which is used by homeopaths to treat neuropathic pain and nerve pain is kava- kava. It is a root found in the South Pacific islands and just like ginseng, it has been used over the centuries for the treatment of neuropathic pain and nerve pain. It is often available in powder and tincture forms for use that is prescribed by the homeopath.

Kava-kava calms all kinds of pain, restlessness, anxiety, insomnia and other muscle tensions. Kava is often used as an alternative to drugs such as benzodiazepines and tricyclic antidepressants. However, do not use kava- kava without a proper consultation with a homeopathic doctor. Also, do not take kava-kava for more than three months as it has caused liver damage, though in very rare cases.

Arnica

Arnica is another herb that is used to cure nerve damage. Arnica is made from the yellow-daisy flower. Its active components are sesquiterpene, lactone, and flavonoids. These active components reduce inflammation, and ease pain and nerve damage.

Apart from these foods and herbs, therapies such as yoga, meditation and acupuncture are being widely used to treat nerve pain and nerve damage. These treatments need to be monitored by those with a high level expertise and care. Herbs and proper prescription medicines can be used side by side as homeopathic remedies take time to show noticeable results.

Section 9

Recipes

Ginger Turmeric Salmon with Spinach Salad

This recipe for Ginger Turmeric Salmon multiplies the anti-inflammatory power of fresh ginger and turmeric powder with the omega-3 rich salmon and antioxidant rich olive oil. Adding salmon to spinach salad makes it a delicious and nutritious meal, which is super easy to prepare too.

Prep Time: 10 minutes Cook Time: 20 minutes

Ingredients for Salmon (Servings: 4)

1-pound salmon fillet

2 teaspoons extra-virgin olive oil

2 teaspoons ground fresh ginger

1 teaspoon turmeric

1 tablespoon honey

1 tablespoon Dijon mustard

Ingredients for Salad

4 cups spinach leaves

4 tablespoons sun-dried tomatoes

2 tablespoons sunflower seeds

Method

1. Preheat oven to 350°F.
2. In a small bowl, blend olive oil, honey, Dijon mustard, turmeric and ginger.

3. Brush salmon fillets evenly with the olive oil mixture. Place in a medium baking dish. Bake for about 20 minutes in the preheated oven.
4. While salmon is cooking, toast the sunflower seeds in a small pan until slightly golden. Now, toss spinach, sun-dried tomatoes and sunflower seeds in a bowl with the remaining olive oil mixture.
5. When fish is cooked all the way through and flaky, take it out and serve with spinach salad.

This recipe contains the following nutrients that are proven to be anti-inflammatory in nature and help in reversing nerve damage.

No.	Nutrients	Food sources
1.	Vitamin B12, B6	Salmon
2.	Vitamin B1	Sunflower Seeds
3.	Vitamin B2	Spinach
4.	Omega-3 fatty acids	Salmon, Olive oil
5.	Potassium & magnesium	Spinach
6.	Antioxidants	Salmon, Spinach, Ginger and Turmeric

Nutrition Facts Servings: 4		
Per Serving		% Daily Value*
Calories	224	
Total Fat	11.6g	15%
Saturated Fat	2.1g	10%
Trans Fat	0g	
Cholesterol	59mg	21%
Sodium	211mg	9%
Potassium	646mg	14%
Total Carb	7.9g	3%
Dietary Fibre	1.2g	4%
Sugars	5.1g	
Protein	24g	
Vitamin A		98%
Vitamin C		15%
Calcium		7%
Iron		13%

*Based on a 2,000-calorie diet. *Recipe analysed at verywell.com.*

Creamy Broccoli-Spinach Flaxseed Soup

This creamy soup provides anti-inflammatory power from antioxidant rich broccoli and spinach, and omega-3 fatty acids rich flaxseed, all of which reputedly help reduce inflammation.

Prep Time: 10 minutes Cook Time: 15 minutes

Ingredients (Servings: 2)

1 tablespoon olive oil

2 garlic cloves, peeled and chopped

1 onion, peeled and chopped

300g broccoli, roughly chopped

1 litre chicken broth

250g baby spinach

2 tablespoons flaxseed

200 ml low-fat milk

Method

1. Heat the oil in a saucepan, add onion and garlic then sauté over medium heat until soft.
2. Add the broccoli and continue cooking for about 5 minutes.
3. Pour in the broth and simmer over low heat for about 10 minutes until the broccoli is tender.
4. Add the spinach and allow it to wilt.
5. Meanwhile, toast the flaxseed in a dry skillet until fragrant.

6. Stir the milk into the soup, bring to a boil and then purée.
7. Season to taste with freshly ground black pepper and a little salt.
8. Pour into soup bowls and garnish with roasted flaxseed.

This recipe contains the following nutrients that are proven to be anti-inflammatory in nature and help in reversing nerve damage.

No.	Nutrients	Food sources
1.	Vitamin B12	Milk
2.	Vitamin B1	Flaxseeds
3.	Vitamin B2, B6	Spinach
4.	Omega-3 fatty acids	Flaxseed, Olive oil
5.	Potassium & magnesium	Spinach
6.	Antioxidants	Spinach, Garlic

Nutrition Facts Servings: 2		
Per Serving		**% Daily Value***
Calories	333	
Total Fat	14.1g	18%
Saturated Fat	2.8g	14%
Trans Fat	0g	
Cholesterol	5mg	2%
Sodium	1811mg	79%
Potassium	1912mg	41%
Total Carb	29.7g	10%
Dietary Fibre	9.8g	35%
Sugars	12.4g	
Protein	23.6g	
Vitamin A		429%
Vitamin C		290%
Calcium		27%
Iron		43%

*Based on a 2,000-calorie diet. *Recipe analysed at verywell.com.*

Walnut Berry Cherry Smoothie

Walnut and berries are the top food sources of antioxidants that help in healing inflammation and related nerve damage. This is a delicious recipe to include these powerhouse foods into your anti-inflammatory diet.

Total Time: 5 minutes

Ingredients (Servings: 2)

1/4 cup uncooked oatmeal

1 cup almond milk

1/2 cup blueberries

1/2 cup frozen sweet cherries

1/4 cup Greek yogurt

2 tablespoons chopped walnuts

4 ice cubes

Method

1. Blend the almond milk and oatmeal until smooth.

2. Add the blueberries, sweet cherries, yogurt, walnuts, and ice, and blend until creamy.

3. Serve immediately.

4. You can top it up with granola or a drizzle of honey.

5. Also, you can keep this all day in the fridge. Though, colour will darken but it will taste delicious.

This recipe contains the following nutrients that are proven to be anti-inflammatory in nature and help in reversing nerve damage.

No.	Nutrients	Food sources
1.	Vitamin B12	Yogurt
2.	Vitamin B2	Almonds
3.	Omega-3 fatty acids	Walnuts
4.	Potassium & magnesium	Oats
5.	Antioxidants	Blueberries, sweet cherries

Nutrition Facts
Servings: 2

Per Serving		% Daily Value*
Calories	182	
Total Fat	7g	9%
Saturated Fat	0.7g	3%
Trans Fat	0g	
Cholesterol	2mg	1%
Sodium	102mg	4%
Potassium	195mg	4%
Total Carb	24.6g	8%
Dietary Fibre	3.4g	12%
Sugars	13.9g	
Protein	6g	
Vitamin A		10%
Vitamin C		14%
Calcium		23%
Iron		8%

*Based on a 2,000-calorie diet. *Recipe analysed at verywell.com.*

Carrot Beet Muffins

These muffins are super healthy and packed with the antioxidant power of beet root and carrot. Flaxseeds further add on the anti-inflammatory omega-3 fatty acids for a delicious and satiating start of the day.

Prep Time: 10 minutes Cook Time: 25 minutes

Ingredients (Serves: 12)

1½ cups all-purpose flour

½ cup whole wheat flour

1 teaspoon baking soda

1 teaspoon baking powder

¾ cup brown sugar

2 teaspoons ground cinnamon

¼ teaspoon salt

¼ cup ground flaxseed

½ teaspoon ground ginger

3 eggs whisked

¾ cup vegetable oil

1 teaspoon vanilla extract

1 cup peeled, grated raw beet

1 cup peeled, grated raw carrot

Method

1. Preheat oven to 400°F. Line a 12-case muffin tray with paper liners or cooking spray.
2. In a large bowl sift together the flour, ground flaxseed, salt, baking soda, baking powder, cinnamon and ginger.
3. In a separate bowl cream sugar and oil on medium speed until light and fluffy.
4. Add whisked eggs, vanilla and grated beetroot and carrot.
5. Gradually pour the dry ingredients into the wet and gently fold the mixture until just combined (don't overmix).
6. Spoon mixture into the 12 greased muffin cases and then sprinkle some flaxseeds powder.
7. Bake for 20-25 minutes, until well risen and golden brown. Test by putting a toothpick into the centre and see if it comes out clean.
8. Remove from the oven and allow to cool for 5-10 minutes before transferring to a wire rack to cool completely.

This recipe contains the following nutrients that are proven to be anti-inflammatory in nature and help in reversing nerve damage.

No.	Nutrients	Food sources
1.	Vitamin B12	Eggs
2.	Vitamin B2	Beetroot
3.	Vitamin B1, Omega-3 fatty acids	Flaxseeds
4.	Potassium & magnesium	Beetroot, carrot
5.	Antioxidants	Beetroot, carrot

Nutrition Facts
Servings: 12

Per Serving		% Daily Value*
Calories	274	
Total Fat	15.8g	20%
Saturated Fat	1.5g	7%
Trans Fat	0.1g	
Cholesterol	41mg	15%
Sodium	191mg	8%
Potassium	202mg	4%
Total Carb	28.8g	10%
Dietary Fibre	2.5g	9%
Sugars	10.6g	
Protein	4.6g	
Vitamin A		53%
Vitamin C		2%
Calcium		4%
Iron		11%

*Based on a 2,000-calorie diet. *Recipe analysed at verywell.com.*

Beet Blueberry Spinach Smoothie

Beet, spinach and berries are rich in vitamin, minerals and antioxidants that help in energizing and rejuvenating your body. Have this nutritious smoothie in the morning to ensure that you start your day on the right note!

Prep time: 10 minutes   Cook time: 5 minutes

Ingredients (Serving: 2)

1 cup Almond milk

½ cup yogurt

1 banana

1 peeled, grated raw beet

1 cup fresh spinach

1 cup blueberries

1 teaspoon fresh ginger

1 tablespoon Flaxseeds

1 tablespoon coconut oil (optional)

Method

1. Put all ingredients in a blender.
2. If you're using frozen fruits, use "pulse mode" a couple of times to get the ingredients moving inside the blender.
3. Then blend on high for 2-3 minutes consistently until smooth.
4. If the smoothie is too thick, simply add some water.
5. Pour into a glass and serve right away. Enjoy!

This recipe contains the following nutrients that are proven to be anti-inflammatory in nature and help in reversing nerve damage.

No.	Nutrients	Food sources
1.	Vitamin B12	Yogurt
2.	Vitamin B2, B6	Spinach, Beet, Almonds
3.	Vitamin B1, Omega-3 fatty acids	Flaxseeds
4.	Potassium & magnesium	Spinach, Beet, Banana
5.	Antioxidants	Spinach, Beet, Blueberries, Ginger, coconut oil

Nutrition Facts Servings: 2		
Per Serving		% Daily Value*
Calories	273	
Total Fat	10.5g	14%
Saturated Fat	6.8g	34%
Trans Fat	0g	
Cholesterol	4mg	1%
Sodium	176mg	8%
Potassium	705mg	15%
Total Carb	39.5g	13%
Dietary Fibre	5.9g	21%
Sugars	26.4g	
Protein	7.2g	
Vitamin A		58%
Vitamin C		39%
Calcium		28%
Iron		18%

*Based on a 2,000-calorie diet. *Recipe analysed at verywell.com.*

Healthy Quinoa Porridge with Walnuts and Blueberries

Quinoa is rich in vitamins and minerals (i.e. potassium and magnesium) and combined with walnut and blueberries in this porridge make a perfect anti-inflammatory recipe to reverse nerve damage.

Ingredients (Servings: 2)

1 cup quinoa

1 cup almond milk

2 tablespoons raisins

½ teaspoon ground cinnamon

1 cup plain yogurt

1 cup fresh or frozen blueberries

1 tablespoon chopped walnuts

2 teaspoons honey

1-1/2 cups water

Method

1. Boil water in a small saucepan and add quinoa. Reduce the heat and simmer for 15 minutes. Stir occasionally, until water is absorbed and quinoa feels soft.
2. Add almond milk, raisins, and cinnamon to cooked quinoa and stir for another 5 minutes, until it is creamy.
3. Serve porridge in bowls and add some yogurt. Top it with chopped walnuts, blueberries and honey.
4. Optionally, you can add some maple syrup instead of honey.

This recipe contains the following nutrients that are proven to be anti-inflammatory in nature and help in reversing nerve damage.

No.	Nutrients	Food sources
1.	Vitamin B12	Yogurt
2.	Vitamin B2, B6	Almonds
3.	Vitamin B1, Omega-3 fatty acids	Walnuts
4.	Potassium & magnesium	Quinoa
5.	Antioxidants	Quinoa, Blueberries, Walnuts

Nutrition Facts Servings: 2		
Per Serving		% Daily Value*
Calories	543	
Total Fat	13.5g	17%
Saturated Fat	3.7g	19%
Trans Fat	0g	
Cholesterol	18mg	6%
Sodium	161mg	7%
Potassium	649mg	14%
Total Carb	89.4g	30%
Dietary Fibre	8.9g	32%
Sugars	28.4g	
Protein	18.8g	
Vitamin A		15%
Vitamin C		20%
Calcium		35%
Iron		30%

*Based on a 2,000-calorie diet. *Recipe analysed at verywell.com.*

Ginger Turmeric Granola

Ginger and turmeric are known for their extraordinary anti-inflammatory powers. In this granola, these are combined with quinoa, oats, berries and some of the healthiest nuts and seeds to make a super nutritious anti-inflammatory recipe for you.

Prep Time 15 minutes   Cook Time 45 minutes

INGREDIENTS (Servings: 5)

3 cups rolled oats

1/4 cup quinoa

1 cup raw chopped walnuts

1/2 cup raw sunflower seeds

3/4 cup dried cranberries

2 tablespoons ground turmeric

1/2 teaspoon ground cinnamon

2 tablespoons ground ginger

1/2 cup maple syrup

1/2 cup coconut oil

1/2 teaspoon fine sea salt

Method

1. Preheat oven to 350°F. Line a large baking tray with parchment paper.
2. In a large bowl toss oats, quinoa, walnuts, sunflower seeds and dried cranberries.
3. Whisk together maple syrup, coconut oil, turmeric, cinnamon, ginger, and sea salt in a saucepan, over low

heat until it becomes smooth. Pour this over the oats mixture and stir until granola is evenly coated.

4. Turn the oats on the lined baking tray and spread it across the pan into a thin layer. Cook for 35 minutes, stirring mixture every 10 minutes, until granola is nice golden brown and has toasted scent.

5. Remove the tray from oven and place it on a cooling rack to allow granola to cool down completely. This will make it crisp and crunchy.

6. Now, break up granola into desired chunks and store it in an airtight container, preferably a glass mason jar for a week.

This recipe contains the following nutrients that are proven to be anti-inflammatory in nature and help in reversing nerve damage.

No.	Nutrients	Food sources
1.	Vitamin B2, B6	Quinoa, Sunflowerseeds
2.	Vitamin B1, Omega-3 fatty acids	Walnuts
3.	Potassium & magnesium	Quinoa
4.	Antioxidants	Ginger, Turmeric, Quinoa, Cranberries, Walnuts

Nutrition Facts
Servings: 5

Per Serving		% Daily Value*
Calories	698	
Total Fat	43.1g	55%
Saturated Fat	20.6g	103%
Trans Fat	0g	
Cholesterol	0mg	0%
Sodium	196mg	9%
Potassium	549mg	12%
Total Carb	66.8g	22%
Dietary Fibre	8.6g	31%
Sugars	19.9g	
Protein	15.1g	
Vitamin A		1%
Vitamin C		2%
Calcium		6%
Iron		29%

*Based on a 2,000-calorie diet. *Recipe analysed at verywell.com.*

Pineapple Cheese Sandwich

Pineapple is rich in fibre, potassium, and vitamin C, all of which help in promoting health and preventing disease. It also has bromelain, an enzyme that helps in reducing inflammation. This anti-inflammatory sandwich recipe, also adds in the antioxidant powers of walnuts and strawberries.

Prep Time: 10 minutes

Ingredients: (Servings: 2)

1 cup finely chopped fresh pineapple

8 tablespoons part-skim ricotta cheese

4 slices whole grain bread

8 large strawberries

4 tablespoons chopped walnuts

Method:

1. In a small bowl, combine pineapple and cheese.
2. Toast the bread for a few seconds so that it does not become hard
3. Then spread the mix evenly on the toasted bread.
4. Top with sliced strawberries and walnuts
5. Serve immediately or wrap in a paper towel to pack for lunch.

This recipe contains the following nutrients that are proven to be anti-inflammatory in nature and help in reversing nerve damage.

No.	Nutrients	Food sources
1.	Vitamin B12	Cheese
1.	Vitamin B2, B6	Whole grain bread
2.	Vitamin B1, Omega-3 fatty acids	Walnuts
3.	Potassium & magnesium	Pineapple
4.	Antioxidants	Pineapple, Strawberries, Walnuts

Nutrition Facts
Servings: 2

Per Serving		% Daily Value*
Calories	376	
Total Fat	16.4g	21%
Saturated Fat	4.1g	20%
Trans Fat	0g	
Cholesterol	19mg	7%
Sodium	380mg	17%
Potassium	359mg	8%
Total Carb	46.1g	15%
Dietary Fibre	7.7g	27%
Sugars	16g	
Protein	17.7g	
Vitamin A		10%
Vitamin C		137%
Calcium		42%
Iron		17%

*Based on a 2,000-calorie diet. *Recipe analysed at verywell.com.*

Fried Eggs and Beans on Toast

Prep Time: 15 minutes Cook Time: 20 minutes

Ingredients (Servings: 4)

3 tablespoons olive oil

1 cup finely chopped onion

2 teaspoons finely chopped garlic

1/2 cup ketchup

2 cans of cannellini beans, drained and rinsed

1/2 cup water

2 teaspoons white wine vinegar

2 teaspoons Dijon mustard

½ cup chopped toasted walnuts

Kosher salt and freshly ground black pepper

4 slices bread, toasted

4 eggs

Method

1. Heat oil in a medium non-stick skillet over medium high heat. Add onions and garlic and cook while stirring, until soft. Add beans, ketchup and water. Stir to combine and bring it to a simmer.

2. In a large bowl, whisk together mustard, vinegar, and 2 tablespoons oil. Add beans and walnuts. Season with salt and pepper. Now, toss to combine.
3. Heat remaining oil in a large non-stick skillet over high heat until shimmering. Crack eggs into oil and reduce heat to medium. Cook, until whites are set but yolks are still runny (about 3 minutes). Season with salt and pepper.
4. Divide toast between 4 plates and serve each portion of beans topped with a fried egg.

This recipe contains the following nutrients that are proven to be anti-inflammatory in nature and help in reversing nerve damage.

No.	Nutrients	Food sources
1.	Vitamin B12	Eggs
1.	Vitamin B2, B6	Whole grain bread
2.	Vitamin B1, Omega-3 fatty acids	Walnuts
3.	Potassium & magnesium	Beans
4.	Antioxidants	Eggs, Beans, Walnuts

Nutrition Facts
Servings: 4

Per Serving		% Daily Value*
Calories	368	
Total Fat	24.9g	32%
Saturated Fat	3.5g	17%
Trans Fat	0g	
Cholesterol	164mg	60%
Sodium	617mg	27%
Potassium	452mg	10%
Total Carb	27.3g	9%
Dietary Fibre	5.1g	18%
Sugars	9g	
Protein	14.5g	
Vitamin A		17%
Vitamin C		12%
Calcium		7%
Iron		15%

*Based on a 2,000-calorie diet. *Recipe analysed at verywell.com.*

Coconut and Turmeric Chia Pudding

This delicious breakfast recipe combines the anti-inflammatory benefits of turmeric with health benefits of chia seeds.

Cook Time   5 minutes

Ingredients (Servings: 2)

2 cups coconut milk

1/2 teaspoon ground turmeric

1/2 teaspoon fresh ginger

1 tablespoon Honey

4 tablespoons chia seeds

Method

1. Put coconut milk in a saucepan and make it a little warm.
2. Blend in turmeric, ginger and maple syrup, until smooth.
3. Bring this mixture to a quick boil and simmer for 2 minutes.
4. Finally, whisk this turmeric milk mixture and chia seeds in a jar, until fully combined.
5. Leave in refrigerator for some time (about an hour), till all the moisture is absorbed or overnight to serve cold for breakfast.

This recipe contains the following nutrients that are proven to be anti-inflammatory in nature and help in reversing nerve damage.

No.	Nutrients	Food sources
1.	Vitamin B1, B2, B6	Chia seeds
2.	Omega-3 fatty acids	Chia seeds
3.	Potassium & magnesium	Chia seeds
4.	Antioxidants	Turmeric, Ginger, Chia seeds

Nutrition Facts
Servings: 2

Per Serving		% Daily Value*
Calories	707	
Total Fat	65.3g	84%
Saturated Fat	50.8g	254%
Trans Fat	0g	
Cholesterol	0mg	0%
Sodium	41mg	2%
Potassium	817mg	17%
Total Carb	30.6g	10%
Dietary Fibre	13.5g	48%
Sugars	16.7g	
Protein	9.6g	
Vitamin A		0%
Vitamin C		12%
Calcium		15%
Iron		32%

*Based on a 2,000-calorie diet. *Recipe analysed at verywell.com.*

Tuna Spinach Frittatas

Preparation 10 minutes   Cook Time 20-25 minutes

Ingredients (Servings: 4)

6 eggs

1 tin of Tuna, chunks, drained

1 tablespoon olive oil

1 red finely diced onion,

1 red finely chopped capsicum

1 cup chopped baby spinach

1/2 cup fresh parsley

1/4 cup reduced fat cheese

Salt and pepper

Method

1. Preheat the grill to medium.
2. In a large bowl, lightly whisk all the eggs together and then stir in parsley, salt, pepper and grated cheese.
3. Heat a large fry pan over medium heat and add olive oil.
4. When oil is warm, add onion and sauté until transparent. Add capsicum, cook for 2-3 minutes and then add spinach before capsicum is soft and allow it to wilt.
5. Add tuna to the cooked veggies in the pan and separate the chunks, gently.

6. Finally, slightly turn up the heat and carefully pour the egg mixture into the fry pan, making sure that it covers all the veggies nicely.
7. Leave the mixture for 3-5 minutes until it starts to solidify. Now, place the pan with set frittata under the preheated grill for 3-5 minutes until the top appears golden brown.
8. Remove from the grill and serve immediately.

This recipe contains the following nutrients that are proven to be anti-inflammatory in nature and help in reversing nerve damage.

No.	Nutrients	Food sources
1.	Vitamin B12	Tuna, Eggs, cheese
2.	Vitamin B6	Tuna, Spinach
3.	Omega-3 fatty acids	Tuna
4.	Vitamin B2, Potassium & magnesium	Spinach, Capsicum, Parsley
5.	Antioxidants	Tuna, Spinach, Eggs, Parsley

Nutrition Facts
Servings: 4

Per Serving		% Daily Value*
Calories	182	
Total Fat	10.9g	14%
Saturated Fat	2.8g	14%
Trans Fat	0g	
Cholesterol	264mg	96%
Sodium	233mg	10%
Potassium	295mg	6%
Total Carb	4.2g	1%
Dietary Fibre	1g	4%
Sugars	1.8g	
Protein	17.2g	
Vitamin A		56%
Vitamin C		23%
Calcium		6%
Iron		11%

*Based on a 2,000-calorie diet. *Recipe analysed at verywell.com.*

Asparagus Garlic Omelette

Ingredients (Servings: 2)

1/2 lb thin asparagus

2 tablespoons olive oil

1 clove minced garlic

1/2 lb sliced mushroom

4 lightly beaten eggs

2 tablespoons ground flax seed

1/4 teaspoon salt, to taste

1 teaspoon minced fresh basil

1/4 teaspoon ground black pepper

2 tablespoons finely grated Parmesan cheese

Method

1. Trim asparagus and cut it into 1-inch pieces; steam it until crisp-tender, about 5 minutes. Drain thoroughly.
2. In a heavy, large, non-stick skillet put 1 tablespoon olive oil over medium-high heat and sauté garlic and mushrooms until moisture has evaporated, about 3 minutes.
3. Add steamed asparagus; sauté until heated through. Remove from pan and keep warm.
4. In a large bowl, whisk eggs, grated Parmesan cheese, flax seed, salt, basil, and pepper.

5. Add remaining olive oil in skillet and swirl it around until it covers the base of the pan evenly.
6. Check when it is hot enough (by dropping a few drops of water), pour in egg mixture.
7. Cook until eggs are very softly set, tilting skillet so eggs coat skillet evenly.
8. As eggs cook, gently run rubber spatula around edges and allow uncooked egg portion to flow underneath, about 4 minutes.
9. When eggs are cooked, place asparagus and mushrooms mix on one side.
10. Tilt skillet and slide omelette out onto plate, folding omelette in half. Serve immediately.

This recipe contains the following nutrients that are proven to be anti-inflammatory in nature and help in reversing nerve damage.

No.	Nutrients	Food sources
1.	Vitamin B12	Eggs, cheese
2.	Vitamin B1, B2, B6	Asparagus, Mushroom
3.	Omega-3 fatty acids	Flax seeds
4.	Potassium & magnesium	Asparagus
5.	Antioxidants	Asparagus, Eggs, Garlic, Mushroom, Flax seeds, Parsley

Nutrition Facts
Servings: 2

Per Serving		% Daily Value*
Calories	382	
Total Fat	28g	36%
Saturated Fat	6.6g	33%
Trans Fat	0.1g	
Cholesterol	332mg	121%
Sodium	655mg	28%
Potassium	817mg	17%
Total Carb	13.3g	4%
Dietary Fibre	6g	21%
Sugars	5.3g	
Protein	24g	
Vitamin A		52%
Vitamin C		19%
Calcium		18%
Iron		55%

*Based on a 2,000-calorie diet. *Recipe analysed at verywell.com.*

Broccoli Kale and Salmon Pasta

Prep time: 15 minutes   Cook time: 20 minutes

Ingredients (Servings: 4)

400gm salmon fillet, chopped

2 shallots, finely chopped

2 garlic cloves, finely chopped

3 tablespoons olive oil

2 heads of broccoli Florets

300gm kale, finely chopped

1 cup tomatoes, chopped

1/4 cup pine nuts, toasted

8 ounces rotini pasta, cooked

2 teaspoons vinegar

2 tablespoons chives, finely chopped

Grated Parmesan cheese

2 tablespoons lemon juice

Salt and pepper to taste

Method

1. Preheat oven to 425°F. Season salmon with one tablespoon each of olive oil and lemon juice. Sprinkle salt and pepper to taste. Bake salmon until it reaches desired degree of doneness (about 12 minutes), let it cool.
2. Meanwhile, put broccoli florets in boiling water, until soft enough. Drain and cut through to break it up.
3. Heat one tablespoon oil in a non-stick pan, add finely chopped shallots and garlic, stir until brown. Add kale, tomatoes and pine nuts, cook until kale is slightly wilted.
4. Now, add pasta, salmon, broccoli, chives, remaining lemon juice and olive oil. Mix gently and cook until heated (about two minutes).
5. Top with Parmesan cheese and serve.

This recipe contains the following nutrients that are proven to be anti-inflammatory in nature and help in reversing nerve damage.

No.	Nutrients	Food sources
1.	Vitamin B12	Salmon
2.	Vitamin B1, B2, B6	Broccoli, Kale
3.	Omega-3 fatty acids	Salmon
4.	Potassium & magnesium	Kale
5.	Antioxidants	Broccoli, Kale, Salmon, Garlic,

Nutrition Facts
Servings: 2

Per Serving		% Daily Value*
Calories	513	
Total Fat	24g	31%
Saturated Fat	3.1g	15%
Trans Fat	0g	
Cholesterol	94mg	34%
Sodium	102mg	4%
Potassium	610mg	13%
Total Carb	44.1g	15%
Dietary Fibre	2.9g	10%
Sugars	2.2g	
Protein	30.7g	
Vitamin A		356%
Vitamin C		178%
Calcium		10%
Iron		25%

*Based on a 2,000-calorie diet. *Recipe analysed at verywell.com.*

Smoked Trout Beetroot Salad

Prep time: 15 minutes

Ingredients (Servings: 2)

120g Spinach leaves

250g small potato, boiled

8-10 radishes, trimmed

175g cooked beetroot, drained

2 smoked trout fillets (125g pack)

1 teaspoon hot horseradish sauce

2 tablespoons low fat crème fraîche

Method

1. Cut potatoes in halves, radishes in quarter and beetroot in wedges.
2. Arrange salad greens on 2 shallow serving dishes. Then divide potatoes, radishes and beetroot between them.
3. Flake the trout into chunky pieces and arrange on top.
4. Mix the horseradish and crème fraîche with 1 tablespoon cold water to make a runny dressing.
5. Season with salt and pepper and pour the dressing over the salad and toss very lightly.

This recipe contains the following nutrients that are proven to be anti-inflammatory in nature and help in reversing nerve damage.

No.	Nutrients	Food sources
1.	Vitamin B12	Trout
2.	Vitamin B1, B2, B6	Potatoes, beetroot, spinach, Radishes
3.	Omega-3 fatty acids	Trout
4.	Potassium & magnesium	Beetroot, potatoes, Spinach, Radishes
5.	Antioxidants	Beetroot, Trout, Spinach

Nutrition Facts
Servings: 2

Per Serving		% Daily Value*
Calories	313	
Total Fat	8.5g	11%
Saturated Fat	3 g	15%
Trans Fat	0g	
Cholesterol	46mg	17%
Sodium	185mg	8%
Potassium	1341mg	29%
Total Carb	37g	12%
Dietary Fibre	5.6g	20%
Sugars	9.6g	
Protein	22g	
Vitamin A		190%
Vitamin C		54%
Calcium		9%
Iron		22%

*Based on a 2,000-calorie diet. *Recipe analysed at verywell.com.*

Sardines Broccoli Spaghetti

Prep Time: 5 minutes   Cook Time: 15 minutes

Ingredients (Servings: 2)

2 tins (120g) Sardines in sunflower oil

150g Spaghetti

150g Broccoli, cut into small florets

2 teaspoons Pine Nuts

2 tablespoons olive oil

1 clove Garlic, crushed

Salt and Black Pepper, to taste

Method

1. Add broccoli in a large pan of boiling salted water (roughly 1 tablespoon salt per 2 litres of water), reduce heat to low and cook for 8-10 min. Then remove broccoli and add spaghetti to the water and cook according to the instructions on the package.
2. Meanwhile, make the sauce. Heat olive oil in a medium frying pan, add garlic and pine nuts and stir over a low heat for 2 minutes.
3. Strain cooked spaghetti and add it with broccoli into the frying pan on top of the garlic and nuts. Stir to coat the pasta, evenly.
4. Add sardines and heat through for a minute, sprinkle salt and pepper, to taste.
5. Finally, stir in 1 tablespoon of olive oil and then serve.

This recipe contains the following nutrients that are proven to be anti-inflammatory in nature and help in reversing nerve damage.

No.	Nutrients	Food sources
1.	Vitamin B12	Sardines
2.	Vitamin B1, B2, B6	Pine nuts, Broccoli
3.	Omega-3 fatty acids	Sardines
4.	Potassium & magnesium	Pine nuts, Broccoli
5.	Antioxidants	Sardines, Pine nuts, Broccoli, Garlic

Nutrition Facts Servings: 2		
Per Serving		**% Daily Value***
Calories	573	
Total Fat	30.6g	39%
Saturated Fat	5.6g	28%
Trans Fat	0g	
Cholesterol	55mg	20%
Sodium	624mg	27%
Potassium	445mg	9%
Total Carb	48g	16%
Dietary Fibre	2.5g	9%
Sugars	1.7g	
Protein	29.3g	
Vitamin A		20%
Vitamin C		136%
Calcium		4%
Iron		19%

*Based on a 2,000-calorie diet. *Recipe analysed at verywell.com.*

Cod in Garlic Turmeric Sauce

Ingredients (Servings: 4)

¼ cup finely chopped onion

2 teaspoons turmeric

1 tablespoon olive oil

1 cup vegetable broth

2 cloves crushed garlic

1 teaspoon honey

2 tablespoons lemon juice

1 cup plain low-fat Greek yogurt

1-pound cod fillets

¼ cup whole wheat flour

Method

1. Heat oil in a medium non-stick skillet, add onion in the heated oil, stir until softened.
2. Now, add turmeric, garlic, honey, lemon juice and vegetable broth and stir for 3 - 4 minutes.
3. Remove the skillet from the heat, whisk in yogurt and then season it with salt and pepper.
4. Heat another large non-stick skillet over medium heat and put some cooking spray.
5. Take cod fillets, cut them into manageable pieces (if too big) and sprinkle salt and pepper. Dredge them in the

flour. Cook each side of cod, until lightly browned, about 3 - 4 minutes (depends on the thickness of fillets).

6. Warm up "garlic turmeric sauce" to serve over cod.

This recipe contains the following nutrients that are proven to be anti-inflammatory in nature and help in reversing nerve damage.

No.	Nutrients	Food sources
1.	Vitamin B12	Cod, yogurt
2.	Omega-3 fatty acids	Cod
3.	Antioxidants	Cod, yogurt, Garlic, Turmeric

Nutrition Facts
Servings: 4

Per Serving		% Daily Value*
Calories	195	
Total Fat	5g	6%
Saturated Fat	1.2g	6%
Trans Fat	0g	
Cholesterol	39mg	14%
Sodium	279mg	12%
Potassium	206mg	4%
Total Carb	9.4g	3%
Dietary Fibre	0.7g	2%
Sugars	7.3g	
Protein	26.4g	
Vitamin A		1%
Vitamin C		9%
Calcium		9%
Iron		4%

*Based on a 2,000-calorie diet. *Recipe analysed at verywell.com.*

Mackerel Beetroot Spinach Salad

Prep: 10 minutes   Cook: 15 minutes

Ingredients (Servings: 4)

450g potato, chopped into bite-size pieces

3 smoked mackerel fillets, skinned

250g pack cooked beetroot

100g Spinach

2 celery sticks, finely sliced

50g walnut pieces

For the dressing

3 tablespoons olive oil

1 tablespoon lemon juice

1 teaspoon Dijon mustard

2 teaspoons creamed horseradish sauce

Method

1. Boil the potatoes for 12-15 minutes until just tender. Meanwhile, flake the mackerel fillets into large pieces and cut the beetroot into bite-size chunks. Drain the potatoes and cool slightly.
2. Make salad dressing by mixing olive oil, lemon juice and Dijon mustard. Season to taste and then mix with horseradish sauce in a salad bowl.
3. Tip in the slightly warm potatoes in the bowl and season.

4. Finally, add spinach, mackerel, beetroot, celery and walnuts, and toss gently.
5. Serve.

This recipe contains the following nutrients that are proven to be anti-inflammatory in nature and help in reversing nerve damage.

No.	Nutrients	Food sources
1.	Vitamin B12	Mackerel
2.	Vitamin B1, B2, B6	Spinach, Beetroot
3.	Omega-3 fatty acids	Walnut, Mackerel
4.	Potassium & magnesium	Spinach, Beetroot
5.	Antioxidants	Mackerel, Walnut, Spinach, Beetroot

Nutrition Facts
Servings: 4

Per Serving		% Daily Value*
Calories	500	
Total Fat	39.2g	50%
Saturated Fat	6.7g	34%
Trans Fat	0g	
Cholesterol	0mg	0%
Sodium	605mg	26%
Potassium	649mg	14%
Total Carb	17.4g	6%
Dietary Fibre	5.1g	18%
Sugars	5.1g	
Protein	20.8g	
Vitamin A		83%
Vitamin C		30%
Calcium		5%
Iron		13%

*Based on a 2,000-calorie diet. *Recipe analysed at verywell.com.*

Black Bean Quinoa Fritters

Prep time: 20 minutes   Cook time: 25 minutes

Ingredients (Servings: 4)

1 cup white quinoa, rinsed and drained

2 cups vegetable stock

¾ cup cauliflower, finely chopped or blended

2 cloves garlic, crushed

4 green onions, trimmed and minced

½ cup Cheddar cheese, shredded

1/2 teaspoon kosher salt

2 cans black beans, drained and rinsed

1 egg, beaten

1/4 cup fresh cilantro, roughly chopped

2 cups bread crumbs

Oil for frying

Method

1. In a saucepan, put quinoa and vegetable stock, over medium-high heat. When it starts boiling, lower the heat, and simmer it for 10 minutes, stirring occasionally.
2. Add cauliflower, garlic, and green onions. Stir and simmer for another 5 minutes, until liquid is absorbed and cauliflower is softened. Add one or two

tablespoons of water if liquid evaporates before cauliflower is done.

3. Now, turn the mixture to a big bowl and stir in cheese and salt. Mix till cheese is fully melted and evenly combined.

4. Add beans and egg. Squash the mixture together, until beans are mostly broken up. Stir in cilantro, cover with plastic wrap and refrigerate for an hour.

5. Spread bread crumbs in a plate and line a cookie sheet with parchment paper.

6. Take about 2 tablespoons of filling in your hand and roll it into a ball, then roll it in bread crumbs. Place these balls on parchment lined sheet.

7. Place the pan in the freezer until the balls are frozen through.

8. Heat 2 inches of oil in a deep-fryer and carefully add some frozen balls. Fry for 10 minutes and then transfer onto a paper towel lined plate, to drain. Serve with your favourite sauce.

This recipe contains the following nutrients that are proven to be anti-inflammatory in nature and help in reversing nerve damage.

No.	Nutrients	Food sources
1.	Vitamin B12	Eggs, cheese
2.	Vitamin B1, B2, B6	Bean, Cauliflower, Quinoa
3.	Omega-3 fatty acids	Eggs
4.	Potassium & magnesium	Bean, Cauliflower, Quinoa, Green onion
5.	Antioxidants	Eggs, Garlic, Bean, Cauliflower, Quinoa

Nutrition Facts
Servings: 4

Per Serving		% Daily Value*
Calories	398	
Total Fat	10.5g	13%
Saturated Fat	5g	25%
Trans Fat	0g	
Cholesterol	56mg	20%
Sodium	1393mg	61%
Potassium	431mg	9%
Total Carb	60.3g	20%
Dietary Fibre	8g	29%
Sugars	5.8g	
Protein	18g	
Vitamin A		16%
Vitamin C		23%
Calcium		19%
Iron		29%

*Based on a 2,000-calorie diet. *Recipe analysed at verywell.com.*

Kale Asparagus and Green Lentil Stew

Prep Time: 10 minutes   Cook Time: 50 minutes

Ingredients (Servings: 4)

1 tablespoon olive oil

1 onion, chopped

2 carrots, chopped

4 cloves garlic, minced

1 tablespoon ginger, freshly minced

4 thyme sprigs

1/2 teaspoon kosher salt

ground black pepper, to taste

crushed red pepper flakes, to taste

1-pound green lentils

1 can diced tomatoes, undrained

3 cups chicken broth

1/2 bunch asparagus, sliced into 1-inch pieces

1 bunch kale, stemmed, washed and coarsely chopped

1 lemon, zested and juiced

Method

1. Heat oil in a heavy soup pot over medium heat. Add onion, sauté until softened. Add carrot, cook, stirring until tender, about 4 minutes.

2. Add garlic, ginger, thyme sprigs, and a pinch of salt, black pepper, and red pepper flakes; cook and stir to coat, 1 minute.
3. Add lentils, tomatoes with their juice, and chicken stock into the above mixture. Bring to a boil, reduce the heat and simmer, until lentils are tender, about 40 minutes.
4. Add asparagus into the simmering lentils, cook until bright green, about 2 minutes. Stir in kale, lemon zest and juice; cook until kale is wilted, about 5 minutes.
5. Taste, adjust seasonings and serve.

This recipe contains the following nutrients that are proven to be anti-inflammatory in nature and help in reversing nerve damage.

No.	Nutrients	Food sources
1.	Vitamin B12	Chicken broth
2.	Vitamin B1, B2, B6	Asparagus, Kale, Green Lentils
4.	Potassium & magnesium	Asparagus, Kale, Tomato, Carrot
5.	Antioxidants	Asparagus, Kale, Tomato, Carrot, Garlic, Ginger, Green Lentils, Chicken broth

Nutrition Facts
Servings: 4

Per Serving		% Daily Value*
Calories	206	
Total Fat	5.3g	7%
Saturated Fat	0.9g	4%
Trans Fat	0g	
Cholesterol	0mg	0%
Sodium	969mg	42%
Potassium	753mg	16%
Total Carb	30.5g	10%
Dietary Fibre	9.5g	34%
Sugars	5.4g	
Protein	11.9g	
Vitamin A		292%
Vitamin C		77%
Calcium		7%
Iron		24%

*Based on a 2,000-calorie diet. *Recipe analysed at verywell.com.*

White Bean Dip

White bean dip is an easy, tasty and healthy appetizer.

Prep time: 20 minutes

Ingredients (Servings: 4)

1 can cannellini beans, drained and rinsed

1 clove garlic, minced

1 small onion, chopped

1 tablespoon fresh lemon juice

3 tablespoons extra virgin olive oil

3 tablespoons parsley leaves, finely chopped

sea salt and black pepper to taste

pinch crushed red pepper flakes

Method

1. Place a small saucepan over medium heat and add a drizzle of olive oil. Add onion and garlic in the hot oil, sauté until onion becomes translucent and soft, about 3 to 4 minutes.
2. Add lentils, cooked onion garlic mix, pepper, salt, red pepper flakes and lemon juice in a food processor. Blend while slowly adding extra virgin olive oil. Blend until smooth and creamy.
3. Add finely chopped parsley and mix thoroughly.

4. Check the seasoning and add extra pepper or salt, if necessary.
5. Transfer to a serving bowl and add an extra drizzle of oil and pinch of black pepper or crushed red pepper flakes.

This recipe contains the following nutrients that are proven to be anti-inflammatory in nature and help in reversing nerve damage.

No.	Nutrients	Food sources
1.	Vitamin B1, B2, B6	Cannellini beans
2.	Omega-3 fatty acids	Olive oil
3.	Potassium & magnesium	Parsley
4.	Antioxidants	Cannellini beans, Garlic, Parsley

Nutrition Facts
Servings: 4

Per Serving		% Daily Value*
Calories	150	
Total Fat	11.1g	14%
Saturated Fat	1.5g	8%
Trans Fat	0g	
Cholesterol	0mg	0%
Sodium	23mg	1%
Potassium	175mg	4%
Total Carb	10.7g	4%
Dietary Fibre	3g	11%
Sugars	0.9g	
Protein	3.4g	
Vitamin A		9%
Vitamin C		12%
Calcium		2%
Iron		6%

*Based on a 2,000-calorie diet. *Recipe analysed at verywell.com.*

Fish Burritos

This recipe combines grilled halibut with beans, salsa, cheese and more to make delicious and healthy burritos.

Ingredients (Servings: 4)

1/4 cup olive oil

1 onion, diced

2 cloves garlic, minced

2 cups white beans, cooked and mashed

1/2 bunch fresh thyme leaves, chopped

2 Italian tomatoes, cored and diced

2 big tomatoes, cored, sliced

3/4 lb halibut fish fillets

1 cup salsa

1/2 cup avocado, peeled, de-seeded, sliced

1/2 cup lettuce leaves

2 tablespoons olive oil

1/2 cup crumbled feta cheese

2 tablespoons lime juice

4 big toasted tortillas

Salt and black pepper, to taste

Method

1. Add oil to a pan and heat it over medium high flame. Sauté the onion for 5 minutes, and then add garlic and half a teaspoon of black pepper and one teaspoon of salt. Turn the heat down and cook it for a couple of minutes. Stir in the beans and cook it until the liquid has evaporated. Stir in the thyme and tomatoes.
2. Preheat the grill to moderate high, coat it with oil and grill the halibut for 4 minutes per side, until firm. Then, cut into half inch chunks.
3. Divide the bean mixture between the tortillas, then put halibut chunks.
4. Mix salsa, avocado, lettuce leaves, lime juice, olive oil and feta cheese together and season to taste.
5. Top fish with this mixture and then fold the tortillas to make cylinder shapes. Serve!

This recipe contains the following nutrients that are proven to be anti-inflammatory in nature and help in reversing nerve damage.

No.	Nutrients	Food sources
1.	Vitamin B12	Halibut, cheese
2.	Vitamin B1, B2, B6	White bean
3.	Omega-3 fatty acids	Halibut
4.	Potassium & magnesium	White bean, Tomatoes, Thyme, Avocado, Lettuce
5.	Antioxidants	Halibut, White bean, Tomatoes, Thyme, Avocado, Lettuce, Garlic

Nutrition Facts
Servings: 4

Per Serving		% Daily Value*
Calories	625	
Total Fat	29.5g	38%
Saturated Fat	6.7g	34%
Trans Fat	0g	
Cholesterol	72mg	26%
Sodium	985mg	43%
Potassium	1149mg	24%
Total Carb	54.4g	18%
Dietary Fibre	11.6g	42%
Sugars	6.9g	
Protein	39.2g	
Vitamin A		39%
Vitamin C		33%
Calcium		22%
Iron		53%

*Based on a 2,000-calorie diet. *Recipe analysed at verywell.com.*

Salmon and Green Peas Risotto

Cook Time: < 30 minutes

Ingredients (Servings: 4)

3 tablespoons olive oil

1 onion, finely diced

1 litre vegetable stock

300 g risotto rice

300 g salmon fillet, skinned, boned and diced

200g green frozen peas

20 g Parmesan cheese, grated

freshly ground black pepper

grated zest of 1 lemon

few sprigs fresh dill, finely chopped

4 tablespoons Dijonnaise, to serve

30 g butter

Salt

Method
1. Pour oil into a wide heavy-based saucepan. Sauté onion, until soft about 3 minutes over moderate heat.
2. Add rice and stir for 2 more minutes to coat well, then put ½ cup of hot vegetable stock. Simmer and stir

regularly while adding more stock, as liquid is absorbed by rice.

3. Stir in peas as well, before all the stock is absorbed. Cook until rice and peas are tender.

4. Meanwhile, preheat a barbecue and cook salmon for 2-3 minutes each side. Then, flake into bite-size pieces.

5. Add salmon to the risotto and stir in the cheese, butter, lemon zest and dill. Season with salt and pepper. Serve and put 1 tablespoon of Dijonnaise on each serving.

This recipe contains the following nutrients that are proven to be anti-inflammatory in nature and help in reversing nerve damage.

No.	Nutrients	Food sources
1.	Vitamin B12	Salmon, cheese
2.	Vitamin B1, B2, B6	Green peas
3.	Omega-3 fatty acids	Salmon
4.	Potassium & magnesium	Green peas
5.	Antioxidants	Salmon, Green peas, Garlic, Dill

Nutrition Facts
Servings: 4

Per Serving		% Daily Value*
Calories	494	
Total Fat	25.8g	33%
Saturated Fat	9.5g	48%
Trans Fat	0g	
Cholesterol	38mg	14%
Sodium	1082mg	47%
Potassium	115mg	2%
Total Carb	44.6g	15%
Dietary Fibre	4.5g	16%
Sugars	6.1g	
Protein	28g	
Vitamin A		61%
Vitamin C		18%
Calcium		5%
Iron		8%

*Based on a 2,000-calorie diet. *Recipe analysed at verywell.com.*

One pot Chicken, Bean and Rice

Prep Time: 20 minutes   Cook Time: 55 minutes

Ingredients (Servings: 4)

3 tablespoons olive oil

1 pinch crushed red pepper flakes

1 large onion

4 -5 cloves garlic, chopped

4 boneless skinless chicken breasts, cut into small pieces

2 teaspoons oregano, separated

2 teaspoons ground cumin, separated

2 cans black beans, drained and rinsed

2 cups frozen bell pepper, coarsely chopped

2 cup canned chopped tomatoes

3 tablespoons balsamic vinegar

3 cups chicken broth

1 1/2 cups white rice

2 oz. (1/2 cup) shredded Cheddar cheese

Salt & pepper

Method

1. In a large pan, heat oil over medium to high heat, add chopped onion, garlic and red pepper flakes, cook until onion is soft and tender.
2. Add chicken and stir for about 3-5 minutes until the chicken has browned a bit.
3. Lower the heat to medium, add 1 teaspoon each of oregano and cumin, and simmer for 1 minute.
4. Add black beans, bell pepper, remaining spices, and balsamic vinegar. Stir and simmer for 30 minutes, uncovered.
5. Meanwhile, bring chicken broth to boil in a pan and add rice. Cover it let it simmer on low heat for about 20 minutes, until rice is tender and fluffy. Keep an eye, in case more water is needed to make rice tender.
6. Sprinkle cheese over bean mixture, cover and let it stand for 1-2 minutes, until cheese is melted.
7. Serve by pouring bean mixture over rice.

This recipe contains the following nutrients that are proven to be anti-inflammatory in nature and help in reversing nerve damage.

No.	Nutrients	Food sources
1.	Vitamin B12	Chicken breast, Cheese
2.	Vitamin B1, B2, B6	Black bean, Rice
3.	Potassium & magnesium	Tomato, Black bean
4.	Antioxidants	Chicken breast, Black bean, Tomato, Garlic

Nutrition Facts Servings: 4		
Per Serving		% Daily Value*
Calories	936	
Total Fat	21.1g	27%
Saturated Fat	7.3g	37%
Trans Fat	0g	
Cholesterol	210mg	76%
Sodium	904mg	39%
Potassium	1941mg	41%
Total Carb	87.8g	29%
Dietary Fibre	10.9g	39%
Sugars	9.4g	
Protein	99.5g	
Vitamin A		69%
Vitamin C		23%
Calcium		16%
Iron		44%

*Based on a 2,000-calorie diet. *Recipe analysed at verywell.com.*

Salmon, Green Peas and Soya Bean salad

This salad is a satisfying and healthy recipe to get your greens, a good dose of protein with healthy fat.

Prep Time: 10 minutes   Cook Time: 15 minutes

Ingredients (Serves: 4)

2 tablespoons extra-virgin olive oil

2 teaspoons Dijon mustard

1 lemon, zest and Juice, plus wedges to serve

1 garlic clove, crushed

400g canned chickpeas, drained

200g frozen soya beans, thawed

250g frozen peas, thawed

100g baby spinach leaves

75g reduced-fat feta, crumbled

4 poached salmon fillets, skin removed

Fresh parsley sprigs, to garnish

Method

1. Whisk together 1tablespoon of the oil, mustard, garlic and lemon juice and zest; season and set aside.
2. Take a large bowl and toss chickpeas, soya beans, peas, spinach and feta.
3. Gently break the salmon into large flakes

4. Put fish on top of salad in the serving plate and drizzle with the dressing.
5. Garnish with parsley and serve.

This recipe contains the following nutrients that are proven to be anti-inflammatory in nature and help in reversing nerve damage.

No.	Nutrients	Food sources
1.	Vitamin B12	Salmon, cheese
2.	Vitamin B1, B2, B6	Chickpea, Soya bean, Green peas
3.	Omega-3 fatty acids	Salmon
4.	Potassium & magnesium	Chickpea, Soya bean, Green peas, Spinach
5.	Antioxidants	Salmon, Chickpea, Soya bean, Green peas, Spinach

Nutrition Facts
Servings: 4

Per Serving		% Daily Value*
Calories	598	
Total Fat	29.5g	38%
Saturated Fat	5.3g	26%
Trans Fat	0g	
Cholesterol	55mg	20%
Sodium	793mg	34%
Potassium	804mg	17%
Total Carb	42.6g	14%
Dietary Fibre	12.9g	46%
Sugars	5.1g	
Protein	41.9g	
Vitamin A		144%
Vitamin C		48%
Calcium		14%
Iron		26%

*Based on a 2,000-calorie diet. *Recipe analysed at verywell.com.*

Sardine, Broccoli and Artichoke Salad

Prep Time: 15 minutes

Ingredients (Servings: 4)

½ cup extra-virgin olive oil

3 tablespoons sherry vinegar

1 large shallot, minced

1 teaspoon Dijon mustard

¾ teaspoon smoked paprika

Salt

Ground pepper

1 cup Baby Spinach

1 cup Romaine Lettuce, shredded

4 oz. Roasted Bell Peppers

1 cup canned artichoke hearts, rinsed

4 cup Broccoli Flower Clusters

4 oz. Sardines in Oil (Canned)

Method

1. Combine oil, vinegar, shallot, mustard, paprika, salt and pepper in a jar.
2. Toss spinach and lettuce together with 2 tablespoons of prepared dressing.

3. Place greens in individual serving bowls and arrange artichokes, broccoli and roasted bell peppers over the greens.
4. Finally put sardines on top and drizzle with another tablespoon of dressing.
5. Season with salt and freshly ground black pepper. Serve.

This recipe contains the following nutrients that are proven to be anti-inflammatory in nature and help in reversing nerve damage.

No.	Nutrients	Food sources
1.	Vitamin B12	Sardine
2.	Vitamin B1, B2, B6	Artichoke, Broccoli, Romaine Lettuce, Spinach
3.	Omega-3 fatty acids	Sardine
4.	Potassium & magnesium	Artichoke, Broccoli, Bell pepper, Romaine Lettuce, Spinach
5.	Antioxidants	Sardine, Artichoke, Broccoli, Bell pepper, Romaine Lettuce, Spinach

Nutrition Facts
Servings: 4

Per Serving		% Daily Value*
Calories	587	
Total Fat	41.1g	53%
Saturated Fat	5.1g	25%
Trans Fat	0g	
Cholesterol	40mg	15%
Sodium	456mg	20%
Potassium	573mg	12%
Total Carb	44.4g	15%
Dietary Fibre	6.9g	25%
Sugars	4.2g	
Protein	14.5g	
Vitamin A		72%
Vitamin C		152%
Calcium		18%
Iron		18%

*Based on a 2,000-calorie diet. *Recipe analysed at verywell.com.*

Tuna Ginger Salad Sandwich

Fresh ginger, lemon grass and fish sauce give this Asian-inspired tuna salad delicious appeal. This salad is refreshing, quick, and super easy to make!

Total Time: 20 minutes

Ingredients: (Servings: 4)

1 can of tuna, well drained

1 tablespoon fresh ginger, grated

2 small shallots, finely minced

1/2 cup red bell pepper, thinly sliced

1 jalapeño pepper, seeded and minced

1/4 cup fresh lime juice

2 tablespoons fish sauce

1 tablespoon vegetable oil

1/4 cup roasted, unsalted peanuts, roughly chopped

sea salt to taste

black pepper

4 sandwich bread slices

Method

1.   Break any large chunks of tuna into smaller pieces.

2. In a large bowl, gently fold all ingredients together. Season
    with salt and pepper to taste.
3. Serve on sandwich bread.

This recipe contains the following nutrients that are proven to be anti-inflammatory in nature and help in reversing nerve damage.

No.	Nutrients	Food sources
1.	Vitamin B12	Tuna
2.	Vitamin B1, B2, B6	Bell Pepper, Peanut
3.	Omega-3 fatty acids	Tuna
4.	Potassium & magnesium	Bell Pepper, Peanut
5.	Antioxidants	Tuna, Ginger, Bell Pepper, Peanut

Nutrition Facts
Servings: 4

Per Serving		% Daily Value*
Calories	241	
Total Fat	11.7g	15%
Saturated Fat	1.9g	10%
Trans Fat	0g	
Cholesterol	14mg	5%
Sodium	869mg	38%
Potassium	244mg	5%
Total Carb	19.1g	6%
Dietary Fibre	1.5g	5%
Sugars	3.5g	
Protein	16.5g	
Vitamin A		21%
Vitamin C		51%
Calcium		9%
Iron		5%

*Based on a 2,000-calorie diet. *Recipe analysed at verywell.com.*

Mackerel Burger

A variety of oily fish can make incredibly succulent patties and with few other ingredients, you can make yourself a tasty healthy burger.

Prep Time: 30 minutes   Cook Time: 5 minutes

Ingredients (Serves: 4)

1 canned mackerel

200 g fresh spinach, chopped

1 spring onions, finely chopped

1 onion, finely chopped

2 teaspoons olive oil

1 lemon, zest and juice

1 egg

1 cup bread crumbs

1 teaspoon Worcestershire sauce

Flour for dusting

4 Hamburger buns

Chili sauce or tartare sauce

Method

1.   Heat oven to 400°F.

2. Stir-fry onion and spring onion in the olive oil for 2 minutes, until soft.
3. In a medium bowl, mix spinach, lemon zest and mackerel flakes.
4. Add onions to the bowl and mix in the egg, breadcrumbs and Worcestershire sauce.
5. Lightly flour the work surface, split mixture into 4 balls and shape each ball into a burger patty.
6. Place them on a baking sheet and bake until lightly browned.
7. Serve in a bun with shreds of lettuce, cucumber and tomato slices and tartare sauce.

This recipe contains the following nutrients that are proven to be anti-inflammatory in nature and help in reversing nerve damage.

No.	Nutrients	Food sources
1.	Vitamin B12	Mackerel, Egg
2.	Vitamin B1, B2, B6	Spinach, Spring Onion
3.	Omega-3 fatty acids	Mackerel
4.	Potassium & magnesium	Spinach, Spring Onion
5.	Antioxidants	Mackerel, Eggs, Spinach, Spring Onion, Lemon

Nutrition Facts
Servings: 4

Per Serving		% Daily Value*
Calories	365	
Total Fat	11.7g	15%
Saturated Fat	2.7g	14%
Trans Fat	0g	
Cholesterol	112mg	41%
Sodium	714mg	31%
Potassium	592mg	13%
Total Carb	35.2g	12%
Dietary Fibre	3.4g	12%
Sugars	3.8g	
Protein	29.6g	
Vitamin A		172%
Vitamin C		42%
Calcium		26%
Iron		27%

*Based on a 2,000-calorie diet. *Recipe analysed at verywell.com.*

Banana Walnut Ginger Ice cream

Prep Time: 5 minutes   Total Time: 4 hours for freezing

Ingredients (Servings: 2)

2 frozen bananas

½ Tablespoon fresh ginger

60g walnuts

½ teaspoon cinnamon

Method

1. Peel and cut the bananas into pieces before putting them in a frost proof container in the freezer for 4 hours.
2. Soak walnuts in a bowl for a couple of hours.
3. Take out frozen banana from the freezer and blend them with ginger and soaked walnuts in a food processor.
4. When ice cream is smooth enough, stir-in cinnamon. Serve immediately.
5. Top it up, as per your likings, with blueberries, cherries, coconut flakes, cacao powder or nibs, hemp seeds, pumpkin seeds!

This recipe contains the following nutrients that are proven to be anti-inflammatory in nature and help in reversing nerve damage.

No.	Nutrients	Food sources
1.	Vitamin B1, B2, B6	Banana, Walnut
2.	Omega-3 fatty acids	Walnut
3.	Potassium & magnesium	Banana, Walnut
4.	Antioxidants	Banana, Walnut, Ginger

Nutrition Facts Servings: 2		
Per Serving		**% Daily Value***
Calories	309	
Total Fat	19.5g	25%
Saturated Fat	1.3g	6%
Trans Fat	0g	
Cholesterol	0mg	0%
Sodium	94mg	4%
Potassium	581mg	12%
Total Carb	30.7g	10%
Dietary Fibre	5.4g	19%
Sugars	14.3g	
Protein	8.5g	
Vitamin A		1%
Vitamin C		29%
Calcium		2%
Iron		17%

*Based on a 2,000-calorie diet. *Recipe analysed at verywell.com.*

Quinoa Crepes with Walnut and Berries

Ingredients (makes 8 small crepes)

2 cups quinoa flour

1/2 teaspoon cinnamon

1/4 teaspoon ground ginger

1 egg

½ cup milk

1 tablespoon maple syrup

½ teaspoon vanilla extract

1 tablespoon olive oil

½ cup walnuts

½ cup blue berries

Method

1. In a medium bowl, mix together quinoa flour, ginger and cinnamon.
2. Whisk egg, milk, maple syrup and vanilla in a small bowl, until well combined. Stir into flour mixture, until smooth.
3. Heat a large non-stick skillet over medium heat and spray lightly with oil.
4. For first crepe, pour a ladle full of the batter into the skillet, and move skillet quickly around in a circular motion to make an even thin layer. Cook crepe on medium high heat until bottom is lightly brown, about 1 minute. Flip crepe over and briefly cook the other side, about 30 seconds.

5. Fold crepe into quarters and transfer to a plate. Repeat with remaining batter.
6. Drizzle some maple syrup and dress with walnut and fresh berries before serving.

This recipe contains the following nutrients that are proven to be anti-inflammatory in nature and help in reversing nerve damage.

No.	Nutrients	Food sources
1.	Vitamin B12	Eggs, Mik
2.	Vitamin B1, B2, B6	Quinoa, Berries
3.	Omega-3 fatty acids	Walnuts
4.	Potassium & magnesium	Quinoa, Berries
5.	Antioxidants	Quinoa, Egg, Walnuts, Berries, Ginger

Nutrition Facts
Servings: 2

Per Serving		% Daily Value*
Calories	470	
Total Fat	29.3g	38%
Saturated Fat	2.7g	14%
Trans Fat	0g	
Cholesterol	83mg	30%
Sodium	73mg	3%
Potassium	344mg	7%
Total Carb	37.1g	12%
Dietary Fibre	5.4g	19%
Sugars	13.3g	
Protein	16.6g	
Vitamin A		9%
Vitamin C		8%
Calcium		10%
Iron		16%

*Based on a 2,000-calorie diet. *Recipe analysed at verywell.com.*

<u>Fruit & Nut Energy Balls</u>

Prep Time: 15 minutes

Ingredients (Servings: 12)

1 ½ cup dried apricots

1/4 cup almonds

1/4 cup walnuts

3+1 tablespoons desiccated coconut, unsweetened

1 tablespoon flaxseeds

1 teaspoon vanilla essence

1 teaspoon cinnamon powder

1/2 cup raisins

METHOD

1. Put all the ingredients together (except vanilla essence) into a food processor and Blend for a few minutes to combine, properly.
2. Add vanilla essence and mix again.
3. Take out the mixture and roll it between your palms into 12 balls.
4. Dust the energy balls in desiccated coconut.
5. You can add 1 or 2 tablespoons of honey to adjust the sweetness. You can store these in an airtight container in the refrigerator for several weeks.

This recipe contains the following nutrients that are proven to be anti-inflammatory in nature and help in reversing nerve damage.

No.	Nutrients	Food sources
1.	Vitamin B1, B2, B6	Almonds
2.	Omega-3 fatty acids	Flax seeds, Walnuts
3.	Potassium & magnesium	Apricots
4.	Antioxidants	Apricots, Almonds, Flax seeds, Walnuts

Nutrition Facts
Servings: 12

Per Serving		% Daily Value*
Calories	90	
Total Fat	5.9g	8%
Saturated Fat	2.9g	15%
Trans Fat	0g	
Cholesterol	0mg	0%
Sodium	3mg	0%
Potassium	154mg	3%
Total Carb	8.9g	3%
Dietary Fibre	2g	7%
Sugars	5.8g	
Protein	1.9g	
Vitamin A		13%
Vitamin C		4%
Calcium		1%
Iron		4%

*Based on a 2,000-calorie diet. *Recipe analysed at verywell.com.*

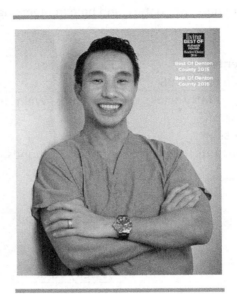

About the Author

Dr. Bao Thai, DC, is a #1 international best-selling author on the topic of nerve damage and has spent over 11 years in healthcare helping patients around the world. Dr. Thai has appeared on ABC, CBS, NBC, and FOX stations around the US and has been featured in magazines and newspapers. Dr. Thai specializes in helping patients find solutions for their nerve problems when conventional treatments fail. He is a devoted father and husband.

Dr. Thai is on a mission to end all nerve damage!

Made in the USA
Monee, IL
31 August 2023